From Bump

A collection of positive birth stories

By Natasha Harding

For Amy - I hope this book offers you something worthwhile!!?!

Natasha xxx

Copyright © 2012 Natasha Harding

The right of Natasha Harding to be identified as the author of the work has been asserted by her in accordance with the Copyright, Designs and Patents Act 1988

Apart from any use permitted under UK copyright law, this publication may only be reproduced, stored, or transmitted in any form, or by any means, with prior permission in writing of the publishers or in the case of reprographic productions, in accordance with the terms of licenses issued by the Copyright Licensing Agency.

Every effort has been made to fulfil requirements with regard to reproducing copyright material. The author and publisher will be glad to rectify any omissions at the earliest opportunity.

Cataloguing in Publication Data is available from the British Library

ISBN 978-0-9572833-0-5

First published in 2012

By Zak Star Productions Ltd

www.zakstarproductions.co.uk

Terminology

Throughout the book some technical terms are used. To make reading easier and more enjoyable here are some definitions of the most common:

Antenatal Groups: Groups for pregnant women in which you learn about labour and the early days of having a baby. There are some offered on the NHS or you can pay to have private classes.

Antenatal Yoga: Yoga classes that are specifically for pregnant women. They are usually suitable for women once they're out of the first trimester.

Cannula: A cannula is a tube that can be inserted into the body, often for the delivery or removal of fluid.

Episiotomy: An episiotomy also known as perineotomy. It is a surgically planned incision on the perineum and the posterior vaginal wall during the second stage of labour. The procedure is performed under a local anaesthetic and is sutured closed after delivery. It's is one of the most common medical procedures performed on women.

Forceps: A surgical instrument that is similar to a pair of tongs. They can be used to assist in the delivery of a baby.

Hypnobirthing: Hypnobirthing is simply hypnosis for birth and can help a woman to stay relaxed and calm during labour.

MIDRS: Midwives Information and Resource Service.

NCT: National Childbirth Trust. Probably the most well-known private antenatal group.

NICE: National Institute for Health and Clinical Excellence. NICE guidance supports healthcare professionals and others to make sure that they care they provide is of the best possible quality and offers the best value for money.

Pessary: A pessary is a small plastic or silicone medical device which is inserted into the vagina or rectum and held in place by the pelvic floor.

Placenta Praevia: Placenta praevia is an obstetric complication in which the placenta is attached to the uterine wall close to or covering the cervix. It can sometimes occur in the later part of the first trimester, but usually during the second of third. It is a leading cause of antepartum haemorrhage (vaginal bleeding) and affects 0.5% of all labours. If you know you have placenta praevia or a low lying placenta and it stays like that you will usually be offered a caesarean section.

SPD: Symphysis Pubis Dysfunction is most commonly associated with pregnancy and childbirth. It is a condition that causes excessive movement of the pubic symphysis, either anterior or lateral, as well as associated pain, possibly because of a misalignment of the pelvis. It is thought to affect up to one in four pregnant women to varying degrees. Incidences of SPD appear to have increased in recent years; it is unclear whether this is because the average maternal age is increasing, or because the condition is being diagnosed more frequently.

TENS: TENS is an acronym for Transcutaneous Electrical Nerve Stimulation, a device that women use in childbirth designed to offer maximum pain relief.

VBAC: Vaginal birth after caesarean.

Ventouse: Ventouse is a vacuum device used to assist the delivery of a baby when the second stage of labour has not progressed adequately. It is often used as an alternative to a forceps delivery and caesarean section. It cannot be used when the baby is in the breech position or for premature births.

Throughout the book there are links to the website www.frombumptobabybook.co.uk so you can see some of the positions mentioned.

Introduction

From Natasha

GIVING birth should be a natural, easy process in a normal, healthy pregnancy but that's often not the case. There is so much fear and doubt surrounding having a baby in the Western World that it's a wonder the human race continues.

Since I began teaching pregnancy yoga in 2006 I've worked with countless women and have been lucky enough to be involved in their special 'pregnancy' journey. I've encountered women who have said they want all the drugs and others who would like a natural homebirth. There is no right or wrong way to have a baby – it's down to the individual and health considerations too.

You certainly don't get a badge of honour by having a baby naturally. However, many women who are able to have a natural labour feel empowered afterwards and my aim is for everyone to feel that way – no matter how they deliver.

Something I've learnt since I've been teaching pregnancy yoga is that a lot of women want to take control of the birth and labour experience but don't know where to begin. I've been in the enviable position of offering help and guidance alongside other professionals and am truly humbled when I hear positive birth stories after the big event.

This book is designed for anyone who is pregnant and who wants childbirth to be as positive as possible whilst still acknowledging that unexpected things can happen, resulting in some women needing medical intervention in order to ensure their health and that of their unborn baby. Many women have a very positive experience after having had an

Acknowledgements

This book wouldn't have happened without the help of so many people.

Thanks to David Grant for reading and re-reading my words, even though he's a squeamish boy! Big thanks to Tamandra Christmas for all her wonderful advice and help.

Thank you to everyone who has contributed pieces to the book; Giselle Green, Dr Pam Spurr, Eliott Green, Mark Woods, Virginia Howes, Dr Helen Terrell, Paula Teakle, Emma Cannon, Mel Smith, Marianne Hale, Lauren Naylor and Erica Davies.

Thanks to Maria Boyle and Jeff Scott, your advice has made all the difference.

A massive thank you to Ricky Oliver for the wonderful jacket cover - and for putting up with me and my changes and questions.

I'm so grateful to all the women who have put pen to paper and shared their very personal stories with me. Without you girls this book wouldn't have happened so thank you, thank you and thank you again.

Finally, thank you to Zak – the inspiration for everything I have written. You are and always will be my beautiful boy.

CONTENTS

Introduction
Acknowledgements
My birth story
Terminology

Part One

I'm pregnant - what now?
What does the average woman think about labour?
The benefits of acupuncture – Emma Cannon
To write or not write a birth plan?
The benefits of pregnancy massage - Marianne Hale
Where will I have my baby?
Who will support me during labour?

Part Two

Labour - the big day finally arrives
The benefits of reflexology in pregnancy, labour and beyond - Mel Smith
Stages of labour
A history lesson
Self help in labour
Women's thoughts that helped them through labour
Hypnosis for birth - Paula Teakle
Too posh to push?
Cardiotocography - Virginia Howes (Kent Midwifery Practice)
Home births
Home births - Virginia Howes (Kent Midwifery Practice)
Birth – Dr Helen Terrell
Being a mum – Gisele Green

Part Three

The Reality
So what does the average woman think about birth and

motherhood?
An Osteopath's account of birth – Richard Whitworth
Succinct birth definitions
Top tips for labour

Part Four

The birth stories
The thing that shaped my birth experience...

Part Five

Let's hear it from the boys
Angus Kennedy
Mark Woods
David Grant

Part Six

The early days
From mum-to-mum

Part Seven

From me to mummy
Changes of a woman

Part Eight

And then there were three
Relationship changes – Eliott Green, Psychotherapist
Baby highs and lows
10 relationship changes – Dr Pam Spurr

Part Nine

Getting me back
Returning to me
Me time – Giselle Green

Part Ten

Perfect mums

Part Eleven

One more step along the world I go

Part Twelve

Glossary

epidural or caesarean because they felt in control at each stage and knew what was going on. That is the way it should be. If you think an epidural will help your birth experience my advice would be to go for it. Make sure you know exactly what it entails – but it's your choice. In France over 90% of women have an epidural – it's just the way it is there and the question is never asked, it's just assumed you will have one.

When a woman becomes a mum she changes, more so than she probably ever dreamed she would. Nothing prepared me for the way I would alter when my son was born.

Our society doesn't readily acknowledge these changes and the end result is many women feel lost when they become a mother. What we all need to realise is often we're feeling the same things as everyone else but nobody ever talks about it. Sometimes just knowing that somebody else has felt exactly the same way as you is enough – it just makes you feel better about yourself to know it's totally normal not to find each and every day of being a mummy enjoyable.

In my experience we're so busy trying to be perfect that we often end up hiding the truth – and yet if you really talk to other women about the way you feel the chances are they've been there and bought the t-shirt.

There have been many times over the years that I've opened up to another mum and learnt that they too have those moments when they feel that everything they're doing is wrong and doubt their child-rearing methods. I can't say how much an honest chat with another mum helps.

I hope this book offers you something worthwhile. I've loved every moment of writing it and I hope you enjoy reading it too.

All the best to you and yours.

Natasha

My Birth Story

My mum died. Suddenly. My best friend, cornerstone and confidante which is how I always thought of my mother, had died, I was just 29, too young to lose my mum surely? Nine months later I discovered I was pregnant and to say I was shocked was an understatement. However, once I got my head around the fact I was going to have a baby I began to see the pregnancy for what it was; a gift.

I had always been scared of the prospect of giving birth and for me it certainly didn't seem natural. At first I thought I'd have a very medical birth – and then I started reading and questioning.

Throughout my pregnancy I was training to become a yoga teacher and was learning more and more about the philosophy of yoga and how it could help with childbirth. I was working at The Sun and had recently taken on the book reviews and was in the lucky position of having countless books to devour.

I took my job of pregnancy very seriously and embarked on it as a project. I read everything I could, played classical music to my bump, did a lot of yoga and spent huge amounts of time talking to my baby. Everything I did felt very instinctive which certainly surprised me. For the first time in my life I began to ponder the miracle of life and to understand how incredible being pregnant was. It was such a shock for me as I'd never felt particularly maternal before.

I didn't have a particularly easy pregnancy. Looking back now I know I was still grieving and I was also commuting to London, both of which took their toll on me. I had a big bleed at 16 weeks and was told I'd probably miscarry and when I had the nuchal scan I was shocked to learn that Zak had a couple of markers indicating a possible heart defect. Thankfully these turned out to be wrong. It could have been quite a stressful, worrying time – but I didn't allow it to be. I remained positive and just trusted that what would be would be – and luckily it was.

I'd decided quite early on I wanted a home birth. I'm not really sure why, but I had read about them and it all seemed so positive. Also, I really don't like hospitals and the thought of giving birth in the exact same place where my mum had been diagnosed with cancer really unsettled me.

My midwife was incredibly supportive about the home birth and her enthusiasm made me more determined – even though there were a lot of people who were rather disapproving, especially as I was quite poorly throughout my pregnancy.

I left work when I was 36 weeks and enjoyed the last five weeks. I met friends for lunch, read, took lots of daytime naps, studied for my yoga exam and sat in the garden. The summer of 2006 was a wonderful one and I savoured every last moment of peace as I knew I'd never be able to relax that way again.

By the time my due date came around I was relaxed about giving birth. I'd had some hypnosis for birth sessions and listened to my CDs every morning and night. I felt totally in control and I knew I had the mental strength for what was ahead.

I trusted I'd go into labour when my body was ready and at 41 weeks exactly I did. Paul was just about to leave for work at 9.00am when my waters went – luckily the sofa I was sitting on was leather and the floor wooden! Because they literally flooded out of me, just as they do in the films.

I was very calm as I knew I had some time ahead of me because I hadn't had a single contraction by the time my waters broke. Also I was doing a piece for The Sun that morning about giving birth naturally which I managed to pull off even though my waters continued to leak throughout the day!

Nothing else happened for the rest of the day so after my photo-shoot and pub lunch (prawn sandwich and a side of fries) - I was able to relax and read my book. It wasn't until 5.00pm that the contractions started and because my waters had already broken they became very intense very quickly.

However being at home and having my wonderful birth partner Abigail (Paul's sister) with me meant I was calm and controlled throughout. I remained active throughout the labour and am convinced that circling my hips and squatting were the things that meant labour was quick and delivery of Zak, relatively easy. He was a big boy 9.5lbs and I did it without any medical help – apart from the gas and air which I loved!

The pushing stage was the hardest work, probably because of Zak's size. I knew I was having a big baby with a large head and I had to work very hard to get him out - I squatted for the second stage of delivery and I don't think I would have been able to push him into the world in any other position. Because I was at home and coping well the midwives were happy to leave me to it which was just wonderful.

At 10.10pm Zak Johnathan Eric Hope was born. For the final push I stood up and roared like a lion – luckily Auntie Abigail was there to catch my little boy!

From the first contraction to delivery it had been a mere five hours and I felt totally empowered by the whole experience. My first thought upon him being born was that I could do that again. Then I tried to walk out of the bathroom and leave them all to it. I felt I'd done my bit and just wanted to lie down!

I was one of the lucky ones. I'd had the birth I'd planned for in my own home and I felt proud and elated. I also had that massive love-rush as soon as my little boy was born – and I was totally unprepared for that.

I can honestly say that having my son has been the best thing that has ever happened to me and I am proud of my role as his mother. I truly and honestly believe that the birth experience really helped me to have such a positive feeling right from the start and I want other women to feel the way I did too.

Part One

I'm pregnant – what now?

If you asked a group of women how they felt when they were pregnant they would probably all say something different. Some women love it and others don't. There are massive changes going on physically and emotionally so it's no wonder everything feels strange.

I didn't particularly look or feel great when I was pregnant. I had eczema under my eyes and felt sick constantly to begin with. Towards the end I had rib pain and such swollen feet and legs they actually hurt when I walked up the stairs. However these minor discomforts didn't really get me down. I think most women feel rough at some stage during their pregnancy and hey if you don't you're lucky so just enjoy 'glowing' and making the likes of me feel mighty jealous!

Every woman carries differently so don't get bump envy. Some women put weight on all over (such as me!). And others have a lovely, neat bump and don't even look pregnant from behind.

My own midwife didn't recognise me when she saw me a week after Zak had been born. My face was totally different when I was expecting because it was so bloated, whereas some women retain their defined cheekbones throughout. Everybody is different and there's no point in getting hung up on the changes.

There are large amounts of hormones circulating in your body which cause many physical changes. Oestrogen to maintain the levels of progesterone and hCG, progesterone to maintain the function of the placenta and to stimulate the growth of breast tissue and hCG to keep progesterone at the correct level. You may feel as though your hormones are taking over your life and you're right – they are! As a result of the changing hormones some women feel moody, weepy and over emotional – it's all totally normal.

For some it's a struggle not being as active as you'd like to be but just remember in the grand scheme of things nine months is hardly any time at all. If possible, embrace the changes in your body and relish that you are creating your very own miracle.

So what does the average woman think about being pregnant?

"I loved being pregnant, my hair and skin looked amazing and I had curves I've never had before." **Lucy**

"My body agrees with being pregnant – which is probably why I've had four children. I feel feminine and full of energy. I also enjoy giving birth and love the early days with a newborn baby. It's something that really fulfils me." **Abi**

"I was so lucky when I was pregnant. I literally glowed. I kept waiting for that yucky feeling that so many women experience but it never happened. I exercised right up until my son was born and was lucky enough to have a wonderful birth too." **Emily**

"Personally I loved being pregnant I have been one of the lucky ones and didn't suffer from sickness or backache. I embraced being pregnant and talked to my bump from the start and loved the fact that I could still endeavour to keep up with the fashion stakes

rather than donning a pair of Uggs and jogging bottoms!! I think because my body was changing I didn't want to feel frumpy but rather went the other way by trying to glam myself up!!! This seems a bit of an unimportant fact to some but it was important for me to feel good about myself." **Bridget**

"I've enjoyed both my pregnancies. I have energy and a general feeling of well-being. I love that special bond that you get with other pregnant women too. It's a special time." **Stacy**

"I had to go to a wedding when I was nine months pregnant. My husband was best man and there I was, looking like a whale with swollen feet and ankles. I couldn't do anything and I really worried I was ruining the day for everyone as I was so miserable and uncomfortable." **Taryn**

"I loved the way my wife looked when she was expecting our children. I loved her curves and found the fact she was carrying our child really sexy." **Tony**

There are many things you can do to make your pregnancy as positive as possible:

- **Eat well.** Make sure your diet is balanced and includes plenty of fruit and vegetables as well as drinking lots of water. Don't buy into eating for two; you only need an additional 300 calories a day. If you gain too much weight you run the risk of developing nasties such as deep vein thrombosis, gestational diabetes and pre-eclampsia.
- **Try to avoid too much junk food.** In a survey that was carried out in 2007 it indicated that women that ate too much junk food during their pregnancy were more likely to have a child with a sweet tooth so try to

avoid too many sweets and the like. Pregnant women need to accept that what they consume doesn't just affect the baby's development while it's in the womb; it actually influences the baby's adult habits. Julie Mennella, a psychobiologist at the Monell Chemical Centre in Philadelphia explains that because amniotic fluid retains the flavours and aromas of the foods, drinks and spices consumed or inhaled by the mother. Because the unborn child's olfactory and taste system are fully functional by the last two trimesters, as early as week 12, the neonate can actually detect these flavours and aromas and develop an affinity that will influence his or her preferences as a baby and beyond.

- **Include the following vitamins and minerals in your diet:**

  Iron is important for blood development and as you need to keep your baby well supplied during pregnancy it's important to eat plenty of red meat, leafy green vegetables, eggs and pulses or beans, wholemeal bread and fortified breakfast cereals. Anaemia is common in pregnancy so if your diet doesn't contain enough iron you may have to have iron tablets which can cause constipation.

  Vitamin D ensures your baby's bones develop properly and also boosts the content of your breast milk which is already being produced during pregnancy. Food sources that are rich in vitamin D include meat, eggs and oily fish. Sunlight is the greatest provider of vitamin D, meaning dark-skinned women and those who cover their skin or don't go outside often are more at risk of vitamin D deficiency, as are those who wear strong sun block.

Calcium is important for the development of teeth and bones. If you're not keen on dairy products, other sources include canned sardines, wholemeal bread, baked beans, almonds and green vegetables. Certain cereals, juices and soy products are fortified with calcium too – but check the labels before buying.
Folic acid is advised for any woman who is planning a baby before conception until the 12th week of pregnancy. Folic acid has been shown to reduce the chance of your baby developing a neural tube defect like spina bifida and therefore it is advisable that you take this supplement and also eat a diet rich in folates. Folate rich foods include green vegetables, brown rice and fortified breakfast cereals.
Omega 3 essential fatty acids are thought to boost your baby's brain and eyesight development. Oily fish is the best source; mackerel, sardines, kippers, salmon or fresh tuna. Canned fish is not as good as most of the "healthy' oils are removed in the canning process. If you don't like fish you can get some omega 3 from nuts and seeds.

- **Exercise daily.** Find something that suits you. Now isn't a time to think about running a marathon or losing weight. You want to maintain your strength and vitality so walk, swim, take up pregnancy yoga or Pilates if possible.

There are many benefits of exercising in pregnancy including:

You'll feel better for it and it can help with body image

It can help you sleep better

It will help keep your weight under control - especially if you are finding it hard to resist the chocolate

It can improve flexibility which may help during labour

It will build muscle tone which may help you regain your pre-pregnancy figure.

However, don't exercise if you have persistent bleeding in the second or third trimester, placenta praevia after 26 weeks gestation, ruptured membranes or pre-eclampsia. If you're in any doubt speak to your midwife or consultant.

- **Do pelvic floor exercises, every day.** Not only will you be grateful afterwards when you can laugh without worrying but some experts believe that a good, strong pelvic floor is necessary for pushing the baby out easily in labour. Every woman should do pelvic floor exercise – every day for the rest of their life and it takes at least six weeks to get the full benefit.

   To do them:

   Tighten the same muscles that you use to stop yourself having a wee mid-flow, pulling up into your vagina. Don't try to pull your tummy in.

   Once you've engaged your muscles try to hold for five seconds and release and then do some simple hold-and-releases, hold-and-releases. Do a combination of the two throughout the day. Ideally find a time of the day when you'll remember to do them – so perhaps while you wait for the kettle to boil, when you're in the car at red traffic lights or watching your favourite programme.

If you're having trouble locating them the easiest position is the sit-up position (on the back, knees flexed, feet flat on the floor). Once you've located how to do them then you can do them standing or leaning forwards while sitting will help.

- **Think about joining an antenatal group.** There are lots of different groups and you should be offered something on the NHS. Different areas call their antenatal groups by different names. There are also lots of private antenatal groups with the NCT (National Childbirth Trust) being the most well-known. Do your research and find one that suits you and your partner. A lot of friends and women I've taught have loved their antenatal groups and have forged some really strong friendships. Many women feel that joining an antenatal group isn't for them as, 'they have enough friends'. However, what I would say is don't underestimate the power of having friendships with women who are going through pregnancy and birth at exactly the same time. If it's not your bag you don't have to do them – but if you choose not to it's even more important to read as much as you can.
- **Read and research.** Knowledge is power and it's important to know what is happening while you're pregnant, in labour and afterwards. Read as much as you can and talk to other mums.
- **Keep a positive mindset.** Talk to women who have had a good birth experience and remind yourself women have been having babies since time began and that many, many people find labour enjoyable.

- **Think about trying some holistic treatments such as acupuncture, reflexology or massage.** Many women swear that these wonderful, nurturing treatments make all the difference to their pregnancy. Obviously make sure that you go to a therapist who is qualified to treat pregnant women and don't be afraid to ask to see copies of insurance and/or qualifications. Don't think of it as a waste of money, more of an investment for you and the baby.

Emma Cannon author of The Baby-Making Bible and Grazia Magazine's go to fertility guru shares her thoughts on pre-birth acupuncture

"Pre-birth acupuncture is a series of acupuncture treatments given in the last few weeks of pregnancy to help prepare the mother for labour. The emphasis of treatment at this stage is to help calm the mother, boost her energy and establish strong contractions.

Acupuncture is inexpensive to give, is safe, normally painless and has proven benefits. I would love to see a day when all women could access it on the NHS as I feel sure it would save money through making labour more efficient and less painful. Obviously there is no such thing as pain free labour but in my experience I see that women have labours that progress well from stage to stage and that they have contractions that are often strong and well established from the outset of labour."

© 2012 Emma Cannon

To write or not write a birth plan?

According to www.nhs.uk "A birth plan is a record of what you would like to happen during your labour and after the birth. The maternity team who care for you during labour will discuss it with you so they know what you want. However, you need to be flexible and prepared to do things differently from your birth plan if complications arise with you or your baby. The maternity team will tell you what they advise in your particular circumstances."

The birth plan is a contentious issue, with some women stating it's better not to bother. I can understand that point of view - if you'd written that you wanted to give birth in candlelight to 'You Lift Me Up' by Westlife while smiling serenely as you effortlessly push your baby out and the reality was you were a screaming, gibbering wreck who started off on pethidine, went on to have an epidural then ended up with a section, a birth plan can end up seeming a tad pointless.

However, my personal belief is that a birth plan focuses your mind on what you do want – and if you've got an idea of what you do want you're surely one step closer to achieving that – but then I am a very 'goal driven' person!

Your midwife may give you a printed form or there may be a couple of pages in your notes. I'd take some time out to picture what you want and why. But of course be realistic too and of course remember that your own health and that of your little one is the most important thing.

Marianne Hale (CIMI) has been practising holistic therapies since 1994 and here she talks about the benefits of massage and using aromatherapy oils in pregnancy

"Massage makes you feel great, and never so much as when you're pregnant.

It gives a wonderful sense of well-being and is a great way to relax during pregnancy which in turn can help with any incidences of insomnia. As you're not able to enjoy certain foods and drinks while you're pregnant it can feel like an extra-special treat.

Massage can help benefit the following symptoms during pregnancy:

- Massage helps to improve blood and lymph circulation, relieve tired aching feet and legs and reduces swelling.
- Many women suffer lower backache particularly later on in their pregnancy due to the increase in the lumbar curve in the spine caused by the extra weight of the baby. Massage in this area will give a huge amount of relief and help tone the muscles which are working with extra to carry.
- It will give stress relief to weight-bearing joints and reduce any sciatic pain.
- Skin can be vulnerable to developing stretch marks during pregnancy due to the rapid changing shape of the baby. Stretch marks are best treated before they arise. In the early months the abdomen should only be massaged lightly. *After four months there are a number of safe oils such as Mandarin and Neroli in a base of rosehip seed oil which can be used to prevent stretch marks around the abdomen and hip area.

- As the baby grows it often responds to the mother's abdomen being massaged. Lively babies often calm to the soothing movement of their mother massaging her abdomen and it is a great way to bond with the unborn child."

Note that:

- It is important to seek a qualified aromatherapist who can blend oils safely for pregnant women
- Pregnancy massage is not recommended during the first trimester because of the hormonal changes occurring in the body during this period
- During the second and third trimester, and even during labour, massage is considered safe and very beneficial.

© 2012 Marianne Hale

"I have always loved having a massage and decided when I was pregnant I would make the time to book one every week as a treat. I found somebody who specialised in pregnancy massage and she came to my house once I was out of the first trimester right until the end. I had a back, neck and shoulder massage. It was absolutely bliss. Occasionally I treated myself to a full body too and having my legs massaged was heavenly. I found it really helped towards the end when I became a bit swollen. Now my daughter has been born I still have regular massages – just not quite as often as I used to sadly."
Nicola

Where will I have my baby?

Pretty early on you'll probably think about where you want to have your baby. Although most women do have their babies in a hospital, there are other choices available and you have the right to choose where your baby is born. Here are some options to think about:

Home

If you have a straightforward easy pregnancy and both you and your unborn baby are well you may want to consider a home birth. About one in every 50 babies is born at home in England. Many women who give birth at home say they feel more relaxed which often means that labour is quicker and easier. If you're having your baby at home you'll have a midwife with you for the start of labour and once you begin pushing she'll ring for someone else to come too. You can also have additional birth partners so you feel supported and comfortable. You need to take into consideration pain relief at home as you won't be able to have an epidural. Most midwives will have gas and air with them but that will probably be your lot.

Many women who choose a home birth will plan for an active labour and/or a water birth. Birthing pools can be bought or hired beforehand.

> *"Having my children at home was the best decision I ever made. I was so relaxed and it was just incredible."* **Alex**

Advantages of having your baby at home:

- You'll be more relaxed and comfortable as you're in your own home
- You will have the same midwife just for you for the duration of your labour, and ideally it will be the same one who you saw during your pregnancy
- You don't need to interrupt your labour to go to hospital
- You won't have to leave any other children (or pets!) if you've got them to go to hospital
- Once you have fully dilated and are ready to push another midwife will come too
- You'll be able to be as active as you like and will have all the space you need to move around as you see fit
- You'll be able to tuck your baby up in its own cot immediately after birth
- You won't have to drink the disgusting tea out of hospital vending machines!

Disadvantages of having your baby at home:

- You may have to deal with other people's negative reactions to your choice
- Even if your pregnancy has been fantastic nobody can ever foresee what will happen in labour
- The only pain relief you can have is gas and air
- You'll have to clean up afterwards!
- You may end up having to go to hospital in an ambulance if labour doesn't go to plan and this could be frightening and disappointing.

Birthing Centre or Midwifery Unit

Birthing centres are only available for low-risk pregnancies. They are often more comfortable than being at hospital and many women find them a good bridge between a home birth and a hospital environment. These units can be part of a main hospital maternity unit or a smaller community hospital – or entirely separate altogether. Because the surroundings are generally more relaxed you may feel more able to cope with labour. In addition you're more likely to be looked after by a midwife that you've got to know during your pregnancy.

> *"I gave birth to my second baby in a birthing centre and it was just amazing. It was like being in a posh hotel. The midwives were just incredible, the room massive and there was so much space. I loved it."*
> **Caroline**

Advantages of having your baby at a birthing centre or midwifery unit:

- Your care will be midwife lead which statistically means less intervention
- You will have access to a birthing pool and be encouraged to use it
- Generally birthing centres are quite relaxed so you won't feel as though you're in hospital
- The midwives that work in these units are very supportive of active labour and will encourage you to help yourself as much as you can.

Disadvantages of having your baby at a birthing centre or midwifery unit:

- You will have limited pain relief – there isn't the option of having an epidural
- You may end up having to go into hospital if things don't go to plan
- Some birthing centres are part of the hospital while others are quite far away.

Hospital

Most women choose to have their baby in hospital. You'll be looked after by midwives but doctors are on hand to help if need be. You still have the right to have the kind of labour that you want and midwives and doctors will provide information about what the hospital can offer. It's definitely worth taking the hospital tour before your due date, so you've got an idea of the layout and the kind of facilities that are on offer to you.

> *"I wanted to have my baby at hospital as I felt safer there but I had a fantastic labour. The midwives were more than happy to leave me to it and I was very active throughout – but they were there when I needed them. The hospital had recently been refurbished and was clean and lovely."* **Jenny**

> **American actress Hilary Duff had her son Luca in hospital and told an American chat show,** *"It was very easy. I went into labour at about 1am and paced the floors at home for about three hours before going to hospital where I had him without any problems at all."*

Advantages of having your baby at hospital:

- You may feel safer which will mean you'll be more relaxed
- You will have direct access to obstetricians, anaesthetists and neonatologists
- There are lots of pain relief options such as an epidural
- There will be a special care baby unit if there are any problems.

Disadvantages of having your baby at hospital:

- Labour often slows down as soon as you arrive at hospital as naturally you feel stressed and tense
- You will be looked after by a different midwife from the one who looked after you during pregnancy. In addition if your labour is long there may be lots of different people involved in your care
- You will hear other women in labour which can be distressing
- You may have to fight your corner for a natural delivery
- You're more likely to have intervention if you're at hospital.

Who Will Support Me During Labour?

Having the right support is vital in labour – it can make all the difference to what happens, so think carefully about the kind of birth you'd like and who will support you the best.

Birthing Partner

Your husband or partner will probably be at the birth as is the norm nowadays - but you may also choose to have your mum or another family member there too. Personally I'm a real advocate of having a female with you and ideally somebody who has been through labour themselves. Before you have your baby it's worthwhile letting your birthing partner(s) know what kind of birth you'd like so that they're able to support you throughout. If there's been anything you've read that has really struck you then get them to read it too.

Doula

A Doula is a labour coach who will offer practical and emotional support to a woman during her pregnancy, in labour and during the first few weeks of motherhood. They're often seen as a bridge between a good friend and a midwife. Depending on their experience they are able to offer a wealth of knowledge and expertise which is non-medical in nature. If you hire a Doula you'll have to do it independently.

Midwife

Midwives are specialists in low-risk pregnancy, childbirth and postpartum. If you're having a home birth you'll fall under the care of a community midwife. Home births fall under the jurisdiction of your usual midwife and you will have been told what to do once you're in labour. For me it was a case of ringing the community team and they sent somebody out, but this may vary according to the area you live in. In an ideal world it will be one of the midwives you've already met during your antenatal appointments – but that's not always the case. When I had Zak, the midwife I'd seen throughout my pregnancy had just gone off duty so somebody else was sent.

If you're having your baby in a hospital you will usually be looked after by a team of midwives unless you're under a consultant and need additional care and help. Again their job is to ensure the safe delivery of your baby – while supporting and looking after you. If you're in hospital it's likely there will be several midwives looking after you.

Independent Midwife

Independent midwives are fully qualified midwives who have chosen to work outside the NHS in a self employed capacity. The legal role of a midwife encompasses the care of a woman and babies during pregnancy, birth and the early weeks of motherhood. If you can afford an independent midwife you will have all your antenatal appointments with her, in addition she will be there for the birth, whether you're planning a home or a hospital birth. Your independent midwife will then be on hand in the early weeks after your baby is born.

Part Two

Labour – the big day finally arrives...

So you've carried your baby for nine months and changed irrevocably. But what happens during birth – and how does your body know when it's time?

Labour is triggered by the hormone Oxytocin which influences the start of the contractions. In this country most women don't go over 42 weeks gestation so if you haven't gone into labour by this stage it is likely that you'll have some kind of medical intervention.

If you want to go into labour naturally – and it is best if you do - there are things you can do to move things along:

Raspberry leaf tea

Many women swear by raspberry leaf tea, which can be taken as a tea or in tablet form once you're in the third trimester. It is thought it may stimulate your uterus and encourage labour. There's mixed research about the effectiveness of the tea – but in my opinion it's worth a try – and certainly won't cause any harm. You can buy it in any health food shop.

Pineapple

Pineapple contains the enzyme bromelain which is thought to help soften your cervix and bring on labour, although there isn't any research to confirm this. Eating large amounts will probably stimulate your tummy, which could also stimulate your uterus. Whether it brings on labour or not, it's one of your five a day and full of vitamins and minerals that are very good for you. However do be careful of having too much as you really don't want an upset tummy during labour.

Squats

Squatting will help your baby descend into the birth canal. It creates more room in your body for your baby to move, ideally into a good birth pose. Squatting can also help to soften the cervix which means when you're in labour it should be quicker. It's important only to squat deeply after 34 weeks and when your midwife has said its okay and you mustn't do it if your baby is in the breech position. My midwife recommended squatting to me once I got to 40 weeks and I did it every day as often as I could. It also allows the back muscles to stretch out and feels great. www.frombumptobabybook.co.uk

Walking

The pressure of your baby's head pressing down on your cervix from the inside could stimulate the release of oxytocin, a hormone which causes contractions. Being upright also encourages your baby to move down onto your cervix. Any exercise releases endorphins so you'll always feel better after a walk – all that fresh air will be good for you and little one too.

Sex

Although you may not fancy it, sex can trigger the release of oxytocin, the hormone which causes contractions. Semen also contains prostaglandins that help ripen the cervix. Having an orgasm could also stimulate your uterus to get labour started. If you can find a position that works, it's worth giving it a try – but don't be alarmed if you don't want to have sex, many women don't.

Mel Smith is a registered member of the Association of Reflexologists and talks about how reflexology can help you during pregnancy, labour and beyond

"Reflexology is the method of applying gentle pressure to the reflex/meridian points on the feet or hands to help clear energy pathways that may become blocked due to the stresses and strains of everyday life. It's safe, pleasant and relaxing; a treatment will provide you with energy as a result of stimulating all the internal systems in your body.

It is non intrusive and safe to have during pregnancy after the first trimester right through and into labour and beyond.

Treatments during pregnancy should be given on a regular basis to gain maximum benefit and ideally you'd have a weekly treatment - especially during the third trimester.

Reflexology can help benefit the following symptoms during pregnancy:

Anaemia, anxiety, appetite regulation, backache, blood pressure regulation (except cases of pre-eclampsia and eclampsia), constipation, haemorrhoids, insomnia, muscular fatigue and tension, morning sickness, oedema and urinary tract problems.

Once you have given birth the body goes through further hormonal and physiological changes. Reflexology can help restore a state of balance and benefit many of the symptoms that you may experience post-pregnancy. It's safe to have after a forceps delivery or caesarean too.

The only problem having postnatal reflexology is finding the time!"

© 2012 Mel Smith

NB: Always check that your reflexologist has trained in maternity reflexology.

> *"I had terribly swollen feet when I was pregnant with my daughter, so much so that they actually hurt. A friend recommended reflexology and I couldn't believe after each session my feet were their normal size again. It was so relaxing that I'd recommend it to every pregnant woman."* **Sam**

> *"I had regular reflexology sessions when I was pregnant and always felt so much better afterwards. By the time I was 41 weeks my midwife started talking about booking me in for an induction which I really didn't want so I booked an emergency treatment in. My waters broke not long after the treatment and I went into labour that night."* **Charlotte**

Medical Induction

Induction will be planned in advance and midwives start to mention it as soon as you're 40 weeks gone. If you haven't gone into labour by 42 weeks you'll be offered an induction. However, make your own choice. You don't have to be induced and as long as you're monitored regularly you may be allowed to go a little longer. You can always try some of the options mentioned to see if things can get going naturally.

The reasons for induction include:

- Your waters have broken but labour hasn't started. Usually women go into labour 24 hours after their waters break but if this doesn't happen there is a risk of infection which is why you may be offered an induction
- If you have diabetes it's recommended that you're offered an induction after 38 weeks of pregnancy
- If you have a condition such as pre-eclampsia that threatens your well-being or the health of your baby.

Some women request an induction, perhaps because their husband is going to be away and doesn't want to miss out on the birth of the baby.

One of the issues about being induced is that the body isn't getting itself ready naturally, therefore when there is a rush of artificial hormones the contractions are often far more intense as they haven't had the chance to build up naturally.

The National Institute for Health and Clinical Excellence (NICE) advises that induced labour is usually more painful than spontaneous labour and when labour is much more painful and intense it is more likely that the baby will become 'distressed'.

According to MIDIRS (Midwives Information and Resource Service) 2008-2010 there is some evidence you are more likely to need forceps or ventouse if you're induced.

What happens during induction?

Sweep

Before formal induction of labour you will be offered a vaginal examination with membrane sweeping to encourage labour to start. This will usually be done twice after 41 weeks. It's not particularly invasive, it's a bit like having a smear test and many women find it's enough to 'get them going'. I had a sweep with Zak at 40 weeks and it was absolutely fine. The most important thing is to just relax and breathe with it – it's good practice for later on!

Pessary

Contractions can be started by inserting a pessary or gel into the vagina, and sometimes both are used. Induction of labour may take a while, particularly if the cervix (the neck of the uterus) needs to be softened with pessaries or gels.

Drips

Sometimes a hormone drip is needed to speed up the labour. Once labour starts, it should proceed normally, but it can sometimes take 24-48 hours to start labour.

Once you're in labour whether you get there naturally or not there are distinct stages. These are:

Latent Stage

Before you're in established labour your cervix is softening and getting ready for you to birth your baby. You may be aware of the occasional tightening (often called Braxton Hicks) and you may have a show (when the plug of mucus sealing your cervix comes away). Some women dilate a couple of centimetres and aren't even aware of it. This is where, if possible, it's good to stay as active as possible before your due date – gentle walking and yoga are more than enough.

First Stage

The first stage is characterised by the onset of regular contractions that become more intense as time passes. The first stage is complete when the cervix is fully dilated to 10cm which will allow the baby's head to pass through. The time that the first stage takes varies with each birth. Many healthcare professionals say that it takes roughly an hour a centimetre but that isn't always the case. Many women progress through the first stage of labour very quickly indeed and there are lots of things you can do to aid the progress such as being active. I dilated incredibly quickly and my midwife was very shocked and many other women have had exactly the same experience. Don't get hung up on this centimetre an hour business.

Second Stage

Once the cervix is fully dilated the second stage can begin. The 'pushing' stage requires a lot of work from the mother and baby too. With every contraction the woman pushes down hard through the birth canal so the baby can exit through the vagina. The baby rotates and the position of its head changes as it passes down the birth canal so that the widest part of its head is in line with the widest part of the mother's pelvis. Once the head has emerged the baby turns again so that the shoulders can come out easily, one after the other. As soon as the baby emerges, the umbilical cord is checked to make sure it is not around the baby's neck, and mucus is cleared from the baby's nose and mouth to aid the baby's breathing. This stage typically lasts up to two hours but for some women the pushing stage can take longer. For me it was definitely the hard part.

Third Stage

Once the baby has been delivered the placenta must also be delivered. After the delivery and once the uterus has contracted the midwife or doctor may gently pull on the cord and ease the placenta out while she places her other hand on the lower abdomen to keep the uterus in place. An injection of Syntometrine may be given to the mother after the baby's head is delivered to make the uterus contract rapidly and the delivery of the placenta quicker and easier.

A history lesson

Believe it or not it's never been such a good time to have a baby. Survival rates are high and hospital wards are (usually) clean.

In times gone by local women helped any female who was in labour. Men weren't allowed anywhere near – even doctors. In fact, in 1522 Dr Wertt of Hamburg dressed in women's clothes so he could assist in a labour room. He was discovered and later burnt at the stake for his troubles. It just shows how times have changed!

Dads didn't come into the labour room until the 1970's and then they were only allowed to watch. It is only in the last 30 years that men have had a more active role and now it's a rarity for a man not to be present at the birth of his child, holding his partner's hand or rubbing her back.

From medieval times to the 17th century midwives were usually in charge. Around this time women often gave birth sitting or squatting. There were various birthing stools available or bricks that the woman would kneel or stand on. A midwife would expect a woman to have 20 contractions before the baby was born once the pushing stage was established. There were many superstitions surrounding labour during this time and if the pushing stage wasn't progressing quickly enough all the women would go round the house opening windows and untying anything they could – a symbolic way of encouraging the cervix to open enough to allow the baby to enter the world.

It wasn't until 1663 that the first recorded instance of a woman lying on her back during labour occurred. Louise de la Valliere, a mistress of King Louis XIV of France gave birth this way – because the King wanted to witness the baby being born – he was allowed to do this as he was King.

Obstructed labour was probably the biggest cause of death for women giving birth before the invention of forceps. Death during childbirth was known as an expected tragedy and something that women were prepared for.

Peter Chamberlen (born 1560-died 1631), a French-born surgeon who moved to London and became obstetrician to Queen Anne, wife of James I invented the first pair of forceps although they were shrouded in secrecy. These weren't ideal as due to their length and shape they couldn't reach a baby that was stuck and assumed that there were no variations in the woman's pelvis.

Later on, William Smellie (1697-1763) invented forceps that followed the line of the maternal pelvis so that forceps could be used even if the baby hadn't descended very far through the birth canal. Forceps had a huge impact on obstetrics as they allowed the baby to be delivered in cases of difficult or obstructed labour. However in the last few decades as caesareans have become more popular and the introduction of the ventouse or vacuum extractor, the use of forceps and thus training has declined.

Caesarean sections started off as very crude affairs. The first record of one was in 1500 when Jacob Nufer, a Swiss pig gelder attempted a caesarean on his wife who had been in labour for days. He'd had help from all the local midwives but nothing could induce her naturally. Not only did his wife and baby survive, she went on to give birth normally to five children – including twins. It is myth that Julius Caesar was born by this method, although caesarean section were performed in Roman times, no classical source records a mother surviving such a delivery.

For a long time caesareans were used as a last resort and weren't expected to save a woman's life. During the Renaissance caesareans became more widely used. One of the first published accounts dates back to 1596 in which Scipione Mercurio stated that you needed four strong assistants to hold the patient down as the incision was made. He then applied a liquid concoction of herbs before removing the baby. We don't know if mother or child survived as this wasn't recorded. Many doctors attempted caesareans during the 1700's to the early 1900's. During this period there was a 50/50 chance of survival for both mother and baby. Hygiene was a big problem and doctors didn't even begin washing their hands until the 1840's so it's not surprising that so many women and their babies died.

The first modern caesarean was performed by German gynaecologist Ferdinand Adolf Kehrer in 1881.

A caesarean section is usually performed when a vaginal delivery would put either the mother or the baby's life in danger. However, in recent years they are also performed upon request for childbirths that could have perhaps been natural. In the 1970's, the caesarean section rate was 4.3% in the UK and 5.5% in the US.

Today, the rate in the UK has risen to 15-25% depending on location. In America the rate is between 20% and 50% depending on the state. Many women choose to have their babies via caesarean section as they think it's an easier option but don't realise they're signing up for major surgery and with it a recovery period afterwards of up to six weeks.

"I thought that having a planned caesarean section was an easy option, without anticipating how little I would be able to do for the first few days in hospital afterwards – just walking to the shower was a mission!" **Lisa**

"I really didn't want to have another caesarean; I'd had two and was determined to have my third child naturally. I knew how hard the recovery was and having two other children would make it even harder." **Lisa L**

"I didn't want my wife to have a section, I'd seen my sister go through it and it sounded horrific and the recovery period seemed so long." **Brian**

"I've had four girls, three naturally and one by caesarean as I had a low-lying placenta. It was actually quite nice to experience having Lucy by section but I much preferred the natural labours. The recovery time after a section is much worse. Also because it was an elective section Lucy was born earlier so she was the smallest of all my girls and she's still so skinny 11 years on." **Abigail**

The UK National Health Service gives the risk of death for the mother having a section as three times that of a vaginal birth. However, it is misleading to directly compare the mortality rates as often women with medical conditions or higher-risk pregnancies often require a section which can distort the mortality figures.

Pain relief

Up until about 150 years ago, the only pain relief available was gritted teeth, herbs and flowers. In the 1800s, Scottish physician and Queen Victoria's doctor James Simpson introduced ether anaesthesia, followed by chloroform, to help with the pain during birth.

In 1853 he gave Queen Victoria chloroform to help her through the birth of her seventh child. The Queen was so delighted she made Simpson a baron.

Nowadays there are a variety of different ways to manage pain during labour.

Self help

If you go into labour demanding drugs and pain relief immediately you don't have anywhere to go. Personally I would say see how much you can cope with as you may surprise yourself. I'm not going to lie. It hurts – but it's all relative. Some women feel the pain very intensely whereas others don't. Honestly!

I never forget visiting my sister-in-law Abigail in hospital just after her third daughter Tabitha was born in 2004. At that point in my life I didn't have any experience of children and had always been a bit frightened of childbirth and babies. Anyway, we walked into Abigail's room and she was sitting up looking absolutely radiant. Given that Tabitha was just hours old I was shocked by this. I looked at her and asked how it was expecting her to say it was awful as you usually hear. I was surprised when she said, "It was brilliant. I really enjoyed pushing her out." For me that was the first positive statement I'd ever heard a woman utter about having a baby and it will always stay with me. Abigail is very practical and determined in everything she does, even in giving birth.

However, if you feel as though you require some help it is your right to have the pain relief that you need so make sure you let the healthcare professionals know. This is when it's important that your birth partner is supportive – and will speak up for you if you don't feel able to.

If you have read up about labour and understand exactly what your body needs to do you will feel in control at each stage. Attending antenatal classes, doing some groups that appeal to you, speaking to other women who have had babies and searching the internet are useful tools. There is a wealth of information available but you have to take the initiative to find it.

It has been said many times that your body has all it needs to have a totally natural, healthy labour. However it may not always feel like that. Here's the science bit:

A labouring woman releases endorphins which are the body's natural pain-killers. Your aim in labour is to make sure you release lots of these; and being calm, breathing correctly and making sure you're in a good position will help this happy hormone to keep on flooding into your body. What you don't want is to release too much adrenaline – the fight or flight hormone. Your body releases this when you're stressed or tense and you will feel pain more. So lots of endorphins and no adrenaline please.

It's also worth remembering that when you're tense mentally you will also tense physically and a tense uterus and cervix isn't ideal when you're in the midst of labour. Think what happens to your shoulders when you're stressed – it's exactly the same as that.

Oxytocin has been called the 'hormone of love and bonding'. In one study oxytocin measured in pregnant mothers during their first trimester predicted the strength of mother-child bonding after birth. Research has also shown that increased levels of oxytocin strongly increase feelings of trust, calm and safety. Oxytocin reduces fear and anxiety and can counteract the increased blood pressure and cortisol associated with stress. When we experience a threatening situation the flight-or-flight response is triggered and the hormone cortisol, mobilising the strength and energy needed to confront or avoid a threat.

This is where the birth plan can come in as you will have an idea of the kind of labour you want and it gives you something to work towards. However, don't be too rigid in your expectations – if you are and things don't go to plan you can end up feeling down and as though you've failed somehow.

If you're planning on having an active birth and if there are positions you want to try in labour it's worth spending time in them before the big day itself. If you're planning on squatting for the second stage for example – but you've never done it in your life before you could have a bit of a job. Remember you need to prepare at every stage and this includes the physical side too. You wouldn't do a marathon without a bit of preparation, and it's the same with labour – if you want to be active you need to do some work beforehand, ideally every day.

You also need to be honest about your partner's capabilities. Paul is very squeamish and because I wanted a home birth I knew that I needed somebody who would support me throughout as I wouldn't have the option of drugs. As much as he wanted to help I knew he wouldn't be able to give me what I needed – and that's not a criticism of him. Enter Paul's sister Abigail who was my birthing partner and the one who supported me – while Paul ran up and down the stairs making tea for everyone and pretty much left me to it. It worked really for us and I actually think having a woman as a birth partner is really useful.

I taught Emily during her first pregnancy and she was simply incredible. She came to yoga twice a week right until the end - and did a lot on her own at home too. In addition she walked and swam.

Here, Emily talks about giving birth to Max

> *"I was seeking publication for a children's book I had written and illustrated as well as conducting research for a one woman play I am writing.*
>
> *I had also become quite concerned that I might have difficulties getting pregnant. It is all rather silly now when I look back on it, but ever since I was a young girl, I had developed paranoia that I would be burdened with just such an affliction. There was no medical or familial reason for this phobia, in fact I come from a highly fertile family, but for some reason I had carried this fear with me.*
>
> *Shortly after my husband and I decided to start trying for a family I suffered severe sharp pains in the area of one of my ovaries for several days followed by several days of heavy spotting which was in the middle of my cycle. This was then followed by a three month gap before my next period. Not having ever experienced anything like this before and haunted by my childhood paranoia, I began to become concerned that there was indeed something wrong. When there*

continued to be yet another break of several months between periods I began to seek medical advice and my doctor booked me in for an ultra sound scan of my ovaries and an appointment at a fertility clinic.

One week before the scan I was pestered by the feeling of bloating and it occurred to me that I should perhaps do a pregnancy test, and low and behold within seconds the test strip displayed a positive result. And so my ovarian scan became my first scan informing me that I was 12 weeks pregnant.

As soon as we decided to start trying for a family I started taking folic acid as well as reducing my alcohol and caffeine intake. As a member of a gym and an owner of a dog I maintained an active lifestyle and a balanced diet. On discovering we were pregnant my husband and I set about clearing out every square inch of our house, including the areas that had quietly been accumulating clutter over the past eight years in order to organise ourselves in body, mind and soul for the new addition to our lives.

There were so many highs while pregnant; the extraordinary sensation of seeing the images of my baby moving on the ultrasound for the very first time, watching my belly grow and revelling in people noticing I was pregnant.

My husband was very excited and supportive of my pregnancy. As someone who had a poorer understanding of biology than a primary school child he strove to educate himself in every aspect of pregnancy and birth, pushing past many moments of feeling sick and dizzy (discussions about water births were a sure fire way to bring on a case of jelly legs with him).

Having grown up in a big family and watching my sisters become mothers, I think I had quite a realistic grasp on what it would be like becoming a mother.

The only thing I have struggled with is getting my milk supply up to the quantities my baby needs. This was not something I realised would be difficult, rather I had assumed that it would automatically flow freely when it was needed and however much was needed. I didn't realise that sometimes you have to work hard at getting the supply up.

The day I went into labour was just amazing; I woke up just after 1am in the morning for a night time pee and upon going back to bed I was aware of a niggling feeling. I lay in bed trying to go back to sleep but after 20 minutes the niggling feeling continued to come in waves so I got up. With the rest of the house still asleep I started to do some yoga positions. The niggling was not painful and so I wasn't sure if I was really going into labour or if it all might pass off. As 6am drew near the contractions had become more frequent and longer I realised that this was indeed the time so I strapped on my TENS machine and woke my husband.

Shortly after that I called the hospital telling them that my contractions were about four minutes apart. When I told them that it was my first pregnancy they didn't seem in much of a rush to have me arrive and they told me to wait until I felt I couldn't handle the contractions any longer before making my way to them, I think I must have sounded too calm.

However after another 30 minutes the contractions were getting closer and although I was not in any real discomfort I felt I should go to the hospital.

When my husband and I arrived the staff, were very busy and didn't seem to be taking me too seriously so asked us to sit in the waiting room. In a sterile grey room with chairs lining the walls my husband and I whiled away an hour with him trying to offer distracting conversation while I stood doing hip rolls and then leaning against the wall doing deep breathing as each contraction came through. The only other people in the room were a couple who arrived at the same time as us booked in to be induced, neither of them said a word the whole time but kept giving us strange sideways glances. She obviously hadn't heard of prenatal yoga!

After an hour I went to the toilet and noticed that something had happened, whether it was the show or waters I wasn't sure. I notified a midwife who then arranged a room for us.

On being examined the midwife informed me I was 6cm. From then on everything went very quickly. I started using the gas and air as well as a birthing pool (which I stayed in right up until the final stage which I found to be very soothing) and after five hours of active labour, and just three hours after arriving at the hospital, my beautiful baby boy came into the world and he hadn't even torn me. I was so jubilant! I had done it!

I had managed to remember all that I had learnt in yoga, stayed calm and focused and had a fast and what seemed an easy birth without the use of drugs (save gas and air)."

Remember the power of the breath at each stage of labour

Over the years the feedback I've had from the women is that the breath is the thing that really helped them in labour. For many it was because it gave them something to focus on and for others it literally took the pain away. A couple of ladies have even been applauded on the use of their breath by their midwives – go girls!

I remember the night I gave birth to Zak. It was a really warm evening and I walked round and round the garden breathing the pain out and getting louder and louder with each contraction. Paul still teases me to this day about my 'marching'.

There is no right and wrong way to breathe during labour. It is the exhalation which manages the pain so practising slow, controlled exhalations throughout your pregnancy is a good idea. When you breathe in this way you reduce your heart rate, encourage full inhalation to maintain optimum oxygen levels for mother and baby and induce a state of calm. These are the reasons why it makes sense to focus on exhalation during labour.

Stacy on the birth of Bruce

> *"I was working full time as a Media Executive for the Kent Messenger and had been planning to have a baby. My partner Mike and I both hit 30 and suddenly wanted to have a baby! It was so bizarre as we were both very social people and enjoyed seeing friends and going out but it just felt as if the time was right and it was the next stage in our life together. We had been together for eight years, so we had done all of*

the crazy nights out, extreme holidays and spending our money on whatever we liked!

It took just over nine months to fall pregnant with Bruce so I feel very blessed.
I did loads of research! I read everything out there to do with pregnancy and becoming a mum, joined my birth group community on BabyCenter so I could talk to other mums-to-be who were experiencing the same, read magazines and watched television programmes like 'One Born Every Minute' and '16 and Pregnant'. I'm a great believer in 'knowledge is power' and I would certainly say this is definitely true in pregnancy.

I also went to pregnancy yoga from 10 weeks and I can 100% confirm that this had a massive impact on my positive experience. Not only did I feel I was having quality time with my unborn baby, I felt that I was doing something good and relaxing. Learning all the positions and breathing really helped with my labour and kept me calm throughout. The other fantastic part about the classes was meeting some lovely girls that are in the same situation as you, and I am still really close to them today. We meet as much as we can and it's so lovely seeing our babies grow up together.

Feeling the baby move inside me was amazing. Words cannot describe it. You immediately bond with your baby as you know that only you can feel it and it is truly magical.

I had a lot of support throughout; my partner Mike was great (most of the time!) but also my friends. I am lucky to have a great network of girlfriends, some with children and some without, so they kept me sane and were there when I needed to moan or vent my frustrations.

There were times when I was overwhelmed by it all, having this little human being totally dependent on me. Also, I was afraid how having him would affect me as a person. I'd heard horror stories about how you 'lose your identity' being a Mum, but I found this to be total rubbish. I feel as though my life is complete now I am a Mummy.

I was induced at 40 weeks, because the doctors thought my baby was too small. I was very lucky because as soon as they induced me I went straight into labour (so I must have been ready to pop).

I remember the first thing I felt was an intense pain in the small of my back, like someone was twisting a nail in the base of my spine. It really hurt as it was constant. If I'm honest, this was the worst part of the whole thing for me! The midwife gave me paracetamol but they soon had me moved to the labour room as it was very clear that I had gone into labour!

Once in the labour room, I sat on a yoga ball and rotated my hips, which helped so much with my contractions. They were coming and going every five minutes. I asked the midwife to put my CD on which was UB40. I found this so relaxing and would recommend to everyone to have your favourite chill out music playing in the background.

My waters broke while I was on the ball, and then the contractions came on thick and fast! I moved to the bed, and my partner Mike said that I seemed to relax more once I had laid down, which surprises me, as I thought I'd want to move around.

Once on the bed, I didn't move. From this point I zoned out into my own little Stacy-world and breathed through every contraction keeping very calm and listening to the background music. I kept saying to myself that with every contraction I was one step closer to meeting my baby. It really helped that I was on a monitor so Mike could see when a contraction was starting and finishing. It went so quickly, hours only felt like minutes, and before I knew it my body was trying to make me push. This was a very bizarre feeling! If you have ever tried one of those machines that is supposed to give you a six pack by strapping jelly pads to your belly, that it exactly what it feels like! At this point I had to go onto gas and air as I wasn't fully dilated so was not allowed to push, but my body wanted to! I LOVED the gas and air; it made me feel so relaxed and helped so much with the contractions. Mike said I even started to sing along to the UB40 CD!!

Then I was told with the next contraction to push... so I pushed. The midwives told me to put my chin to my chest and make no noise and push. My baby's heartbeat dropped a bit so the doctor told me she was going to give me an episiotomy (a cut) to help him out and they also used a ventouse (a cap that it put on the baby's head to help pull him out) after another two pushes my son was born!

Because I had no pain relief, I knew everything that was happening and could feel everything. I felt his head come out, his shoulders, his body then his legs. I could physically feel him leave my body and enter the world, all 7lb 2oz of him. It was amazing; I can definitely say that I 'gave birth'.

I felt an enormous sense of relief, especially when he cried because I knew he was okay. They gave him to me and I remember looking down at him and thinking... wow, you're my son and I love you."

One word of caution is this though... I've heard from many women over the years that have been so calm because they've nailed the breathing techniques that their midwife wasn't aware they were in established labour. If you've been practising your breath work throughout your pregnancy and in the early stages of labour it's well worth letting your midwife know. Some women catch their midwife out with their calm demeanour so make sure you stand your ground – listen to your body and trust your instincts.

Early Stages of Labour

If you can, spend some time alone at the start of labour to prepare yourself for the task ahead. Perhaps you could do some breath work or a positive visualisation.

Breathing exercises for the start of labour:

Time out breath

Sit or lie down in a comfortable position; make sure you're comfortable as you're going to be here for the next five minutes or so – don't forget to turn off your phone!

Place your hands on your tummy and allow your breath to find its own natural path. Become aware of cool air as you breathe in through your nose and warm air as you breathe out through your nose.

Don't force the breath to be slow; allow it to find its own natural path.

Once your breath feels slow and relaxed you're going to simply count backwards from 20 to zero. As you do this, you don't hold your breath at any time, you just breathe at your own natural pace and rhythm.

To begin... Breathe in start counting from 20, breathe out, count down to 19, breathe in 18, and breathe out 17... Continue in this fashion until zero. Observe any changes in your body and mind – if you've got the time and inclination you might do it again.

Visualisation during labour (for the early stages)

Sit or lie in a comfortable position. The breath should become the focal point - observe the breath as it enters and leaves your body. Whilst watching the breath - picture the whole of your body. Imagine the clothes you're wearing, the way you're lying - picture every detail. Now focus on your body and watch the ribcage expand with every breath that you take.

Begin to colour the breath white. See the lungs filling with a beautiful white light and emptying again. Picture the stream of light entering and leaving the body. Awareness should now be brought to the blood stream. Visualise the blood delivering white light to every cell in the body. The blood then returns to the lungs so that the white light leaves the body and the cycle continues. White light passes in and out through the nose, travelling through the entire body - feeding every cell. As every cell is touched with white light so it relaxes.

The feet relax, so do the ankles, the calves, the knees, the thighs, the pelvis, the uterus, enabling the baby to eventually leave the body without too many restrictions. The abdomen relaxes, then the chest, the shoulders, the neck, the face, the head and the whole body.

Place your hands on your abdomen and direct the white light to the baby with love and warmth. Maintain the image for a while, talk to your baby, do and say whatever feels right and necessary for you. When the time is right then let the image subside.

Once you've finished your breath work and/or visualisation allow your breath to return to normal, roll your shoulders and gently rise. Your baby is on its way!

Labour breath

Focussing on your breathing will help maintain a healthy flow of positive energy entering the body and mind. On the exhalation you should try and release tension from the body. Literally let it go... These techniques should feel like second nature if you've been practising them before your due date.

Once the contractions start building keep your breath as a focus. Gently breathe in through your nose and sigh as you breathe out – become louder if you feel you need to. This sighing breath is great for the first stage of labour.

Ha breath

Once the contractions begin you may want to step the breath up. Many women find the ha breath can be a Godsend. It also gives you something to focus on rather than the pain itself. The ha breath can be used in the first stage of labour, but many women would rather use the sighing breath to begin with and then step up to the ha breath as the contractions become stronger.

For the ha breath: Inhale deeply through the nose and exhale slowly through the mouth making a long, drawn out sound of haaaa. The exhalation should be timed with the most painful part of the contraction and last the remaining duration of the contraction. Use the ha breath according to the contractions, for example, in the beginning when the contractions are more manageable your ha breath is softer and more of a heavy sigh. Once things step up the ha breath becomes louder and more drawn out.

Make sure you rest in between the contractions. Allow your breath to return to normal – in through the nose and out through the nose if possible. This allows you to calm down and have some rest before the next contraction.

> *"I think the whole hospital must have heard my 'ha' breaths, but it really did give me something to focus on."* **Karen**

Jenny shares her experiences on her second baby's birth – and how it was so much better than the first

> *"I'd had a show and been having cramps all day but was convinced that nothing was going to be happening anytime soon as my due date was six days away and my first daughter Freya had been so overdue (12 days).*
>
> *My Mum and family came round in the evening and she insisted on taking Freya home with her even though I kept saying nothing was going to happen!*
>
> *I'd had mild pains all day, but they started getting stronger so I started doing my breathing exercises and at 11pm the contractions were really regular. I put the TENS machine on and carried on with the breathing and at 12.30am, my husband Dave insisted on going to hospital but I was still convinced it was going to be ages.*
>
> *We got to the hospital at 1am and my waters broke in the car park. I was still in denial though and when I was examined couldn't believe it when the midwife said I was 8cm dilated! I got in the pool at half one and twenty five minutes later with only two pushes, she was out!*
>
> *I put all this down to the yoga and all the breathing exercises I had learnt. I was on all fours when the*

contractions came and it helped so much, I cannot believe how quick it all was.

It was a much more positive experience than my first labour and Dave said I was like a different person this time. I felt so much more in control. The midwife said that Heidi was in an excellent birth position too unlike Freya who was back to back.

Throughout the whole process I was so calm – the breathing definitely helped."

Positive affirmations in labour

Many women choose their own mantra or affirmation for labour, something that they know will drive them through.

It may be something such as, "every single contraction I have means I'm closer to meeting my baby." Or "I can do this" or simply "my body is amazing". It doesn't matter what it is – if it works for you, it's worth doing. It may be worth telling your birth partner that you'd like to use a positive affirmation or mantra so they can say it with you – or remind you of it if things become hard.

At some point in every labour there will be a point where you don't think you can do it – this is where having a good partner is imperative. Reflecting on Zak's birth there was a moment when I'd been pushing for a long time and just didn't think I had it in me to continue. I could hear the midwives begin to mutter about not letting me go too much longer – then Abigail crouched down beside me and whispered in my ear, "Come on, this is what you've been waiting for all this time." Those words combined with my own determination about not having to deliver in hospital were enough to spur me on – and not long after Zak was born. The power of the mind is hugely important – and I've said often that my mind birthed my baby rather than anything else.

So what was helpful during labour?

> *"I focused on my older daughter's face the whole time when I was in labour with my second child, it really helped."* **Zoe**

> *"My husband counted the time each contraction was taking and it was incredibly useful. I'd read somewhere that they shouldn't last longer than 60 seconds so hearing him countdown made it much more bearable."* **Liz**

Active Positions

Being active and upright can make labour shorter and much less painful. Being upright also makes your contractions more efficient. Many women find kneeling and leaning forwards help especially if your back is aching. Some women swear by the birthing ball and others find squats and hip rolling help the most. There are some women who reckon stair walking(!) was the thing that helped the most and others found sitting on the toilet throughout labour made a difference. One woman was advised by her midwife to stand in the door frame with her legs wide and her arms up – just like a star. A lot of maternity units have ropes dangling from the ceiling so women can hang on to them. It really doesn't matter what it is as long as it helps YOU.

Personally I think moving is a great distraction. If you're just lying on the bed you're almost waiting for the next contraction to come and the discomfort that comes with it. Moving around will give you a focus.

The positions that have had the most positive feedback in my experience are:

- Hands and knees or elbows and knees
- Hip rolling, either when standing up or sitting on a birthing ball
- Squatting
- Standing or walking
- Leaning forwards and either holding on to a birthing ball or the bed.

Remember when you move you will release those ever-important endorphins which will help with the pain.

Lucy on giving birth to Dylan

> *"Before I fell pregnant I was running a Dance School. I was teaching 38 hours a week and running the administrative side of the school as well as working on a new project.*
>
> *I had only moved in with my then partner three months before I found out I was pregnant so we were still very much getting settled ourselves in our new home. I was busy!*
>
> *Although we'd spoken about having children it wasn't planned.*
>
> *I attended a weekly antenatal yoga class as well as keeping all of my dance classes going. I only dropped ballet from my schedule two months before I had my son. I also swam twice a week, and went to a hypnobirthing specialist for three sessions and listened to the CDs provided every night before I went to bed from about 25 weeks onwards. There were some great times. I felt incredible (once the nausea had passed!) and overall I loved being pregnant. It was the ultimate experience in feeling feminine. I glowed and it suited me. The second trimester was*

the best I have ever felt in my life. I had shiny thick hair and beautiful skin and nails. My mum was a star while I was pregnant; she whisked me away to the Isle of Wight for a week when I was about 13 weeks, cooked me meals, brought me extra jumpers when I was cold and opened windows when I was too hot.

At 8.30pm on the 12th February 2010 I taught my final class of the term, thus commencing five weeks off before I was due to give birth. At 8.30am on the 13th February 2010 my waters broke and I went into labour.

When I got to hospital there were no beds in the labour ward so I was put straight into the delivery suite. They didn't think I was in established labour as I was in such control, until they examined me and I was 7cm dilated.

For the next couple of hours I focused on my breathing and just let my body take over. Then, suddenly, I had the first sensation of pushing; totally involuntary stomach ripples that I could feel were squeezing Dylan out towards the world. We buzzed and the midwife came in.

She explained the second phase of labour to me, examined me and I was indeed fully dilated and the baby was starting to move down the birth canal. This was really exciting and by this stage the pain was totally different. It was a bit like (though obviously more intense!) having a wobbly tooth, it hurts but you're compelled to wiggle it a bit anyway. I felt able to get behind each contraction and push. By this stage I had been in labour for about eight hours and had spent the vast majority of it in various yoga poses and the whole of it focusing on a steady climb up a hill and back down again amongst other techniques like turning the pain dial down. It really worked for me. I felt in control of what was happening to my body even though the midwife was repeatedly changing throughout.

The last four hours of pushing were hard. I ended up kneeling over the back of the bed, but I was starting to tire. I'd eaten at 9pm the night before but it was more of a snack than a dinner, I'd been unable to keep my breakfast down and I was feeling weak and heady at the lack of sugar in my system. I had some Lucozade which gave me a much-needed boost. I then decided to try being on my back for a while which slowed the labour and to be honest got me into a bit of a pickle.

After an hour in this position I could reach down and feel the top of Dylan's head arriving at the end of the birth canal and I was so excited it spurred me on to push and stay on that push until the next contraction and then in one incredible split second there he was.

He slithered out into the world looking like a wet jellyfish with a slightly blue tinge. For that split second I held my breath, I looked at him in the midwife's hands in total disbelief and anticipation... and then... 'waaaaaaahh', he opened his lungs for the first time and started to breathe.

It was in that split second that the love flooded in. I felt my whole world change and I will never ever forget that moment as long as I live.

I waited the half an hour or so for the next contraction to deliver the placenta naturally and was delighted to have achieved my personal goal of not having any pain relief or gas and air. I was also very pleased not to have had an episiotomy or any tearing.

> I delivered at 35wks and two days, my premature baby weighed in at 7lb 1oz - I don't think the last part of the story would have been quite the same if I had gone full term, I think I'd have delivered a giant!! It was about 30 seconds after he'd been born that the midwife asked if 'baby' had a name, I realised I didn't know what I'd had, a quick glance down and I realised that I had a little boy. He was from that moment on officially Dylan."

Lying down in labour is not recommended. If you're flat on your back gravity can't assist with pushing your baby through the birth canal or to help your cervix dilate. The following are disadvantages of lying down:

- More painful contractions
- Less effective contractions
- Longer labour
- Reduced blood flow to your baby
- Smaller passage through the pelvis for your baby.

If you have to lie on your bed to be monitored the breath becomes even more important. However, don't be bullied by your midwife – tell them from the start you want to be active and make sure they explain why you can't be monitored while you're standing or moving. Make sure you're fully informed at each and every stage.

If possible, lie on your left side or get the midwife to adjust the bed so your back is supported by lots of pillows and you can have the soles of your feet together and allow your knees to drop to the side. This position is called Supta Baddakonasana (supine cobbler) in yoga and is very beneficial in labour as you're creating lots of room for the baby.

www.frombumptobabybook.co.uk

If you are getting tired, lying on your left side is a good option. It enables you to have a much needed rest, can slow a fast moving delivery. It gives the baby the maximum amount of oxygen and it helps the baby to still be able to move through the pelvis.

Hydrotherapy

Water can help you relax and make the contractions seem less painful. Both the Royal College of Obstetricians and Gynaecologists and the Royal College of Midwives support labouring in water for healthy women with uncomplicated pregnancies. The evidence to support underwater birth is less clear but complications are rare. However, many women say their labour was almost painless by having their baby in water. One thing to remember is it can slow labour down so speak to your midwife about the best time to go into the water.

Caroline's daughter Ruth was born in water

> *"I had recently got married and moved from London to Kent. We were really happy and planned to have children. When we realised I was expecting we decorated the nursery and bought lots of equipment – we didn't go mad though!*
>
> *With regard to preparing for the birth, we had thought about this from the beginning of the pregnancy. Six years before falling pregnant I had a hip replacement and was told by my consultant that I may well end up bedridden for the majority of my pregnancy. I was absolutely determined that this wouldn't be the case – I am not a sit around and do nothing type of person!*
>
> *From 12 weeks, I started pregnancy yoga. This was the best decision (other than choosing to fall pregnant!) that I made. It helped me so much. I did have some problems with my hip and SPD (Symphysis Pubis Dysfunction) but I even went to yoga when I was walking with crutches for a couple of weeks. Yoga helped with my hip, kept me out of bed and made me stronger physically for the birth. I felt empowered and incredibly determined that I would be able to get through the pregnancy as well as having*

an active birth – I couldn't think of anything worse than having a caesarean, not least because you're not allowed to drive for so long afterwards. I didn't want my independence taken away.

Being new to the area, I also knew very few people, let alone anyone with a baby, so we joined the NCT, did their antenatal course and met a fabulous group of people – and have subsequently stayed in touch with all of them.

Leaving work was incredibly strange. I am a teacher and I remember the first day of maternity leave thinking about what the children would be doing – that soon passed though!

It was also emotional when the first couple in our NCT group gave birth to their baby. I remember wanting to know all the details but restraining myself and giving them the time that they needed and deserved!

When the day finally arrived for me the contractions started on Tuesday evening. I keep thinking back to how it all began but can't actually remember when I realised that I was contracting. My husband found my TENS machine and plugged me in! The contractions were very irregular and so we went to bed as usual and then they stopped completely in the morning!

Wednesday was a strange day. We kept looking at each other not really knowing what to do. We went out for a walk, not too far so that we could pop home if needed. The contractions started again that evening, but again, nothing regular and so we slept well that evening too.

Thursday morning the contractions were also irregular and not very powerful, so we pottered around the house a little and did some yoga together, until about 3pm when they started to become more regular.

My husband called the hospital at about 5pm, as he wanted to let someone know what was happening and to check that everything was okay. I spoke to a midwife who said I sounded very calm and that it wasn't time to come in yet and that I would know when they right time would be.

About five minutes after hanging up, I asked my husband to call them back as I wanted to go in. He wasn't too keen as he didn't want to be a pain, but rang anyway. The maternity unit said that they were quiet so we could go in, but we should be prepared to be sent home.

Being the determined lady that I am, I insisted upon walking up the stairs to the delivery suite – it wasn't easy and took a little while! We were greeted by a midwife.

By now the contractions were strong and regular, but the TENS machine was fabulous, as was the breathing that I learnt in yoga. The midwife looked at me and said "I doubt if you'll stay here long, you are too calm to be in established labour!" Famous last words!

I was examined and told that I was about 5cm, so I could go in the birthing pool if I wanted, but I was likely to be in there a long time. Not long after the midwife had left the room, I was sick. This was no surprise to me or my husband as I had been sick throughout pregnancy so why should now be any different? Whilst being sick I also burst my waters – whoever said that there was nothing attractive about giving birth was right!

I got myself cleaned up and then down the corridor into the birthing pool. The water was lovely, but I didn't like taking the TENS machine off. I climbed into the pool at 8:10pm. After about 15 minutes I told the midwife that I wanted to push. She told me that I wasn't ready.

My husband whispered in my ear, "If you want to push then you push!" I will remember those words forever! The next contraction I pushed and felt pressure. My husband looked in the water and said "Is that normal?" Now these are not words any lady in labour wants to hear and so in the split second that it took the midwife to reply all sorts of crazy ideas were going through my head. "Wow" she said "That's the head!" The next minute or two were a bit of a blur as the midwife wasn't fully prepared. I remember hearing that the water wasn't the right temperature for the baby and another midwife or two running into the room with all sorts of things.

The next contraction came and I birthed my baby, the midwife helped me bring her to the surface of the water, and I flipped her over to discover that she was indeed a girl!

It was the most delightful and amazing moment. Just thinking about it brings a tear to my eye. We stayed in the water for a while and the three of us just cuddled and felt like a little family for the first time. Blissful! I was shocked and amazed all in one go.

During the birth my husband was with me throughout. He likes having a job to do, so he started timing the contractions. Once I was in early labour I discovered the best breathing for me and showed it to my husband. He then reminded me of this during established labour. He also gave me the strength and encouragement that I needed and kept telling me that

> I could do it. Giving birth was just wonderful and I wouldn't change a thing."

TENS

TENS is an acronym for Transcutaneous Electrical Nerve Stimulation machines. Some hospitals have TENS machines or you can hire your own. I would recommend this as it gives you some time to play around with it before the big day. They have been shown to be most effective during the early stages of labour and during home births where pain relief options are more limited. Some women find them very useful in the early stages of labour and then get a bit aggravated by them after a while. If you're planning on using one, it's worth making sure you know how to use it well in advance and that you have enough batteries. I used a TENS machine and it was really useful for the majority of the time, until I got fed up with it and ripped it off me. I've since heard that's quite common!

Nicola on the birth of Olivia

> "When I found out I was pregnant despite it being something we had wanted for a long time I burst into tears because I was absolutely terrified. Once I got over that initial reaction I felt very excited and absolutely loved being pregnant.
>
> I prepared well for the birth in terms of antenatal classes, yoga and hypnobirthing as I was frightened of the prospect of giving birth and wanted to deal with that issue properly.
>
> The best advice I had was to remember to give into your natural instincts. I remember the midwife at the

antenatal class telling us to 'act like animals do in labour' – bizarre but so sensible.

I had a few fears while I was pregnant. I was afraid of not being around for my child in years to come having lost my mother at a young age. It was not until she was born that I was hit one day with this absolute feeling of terror of how I would ever cope if I lost her.

I finally went into labour when I was over two weeks overdue and getting frustrated. The first sign was mild contractions that started just after midnight. I got up and sat on a gym ball (the only comfortable position I had found at the end of the pregnancy) and watched TV and read a Harry Potter adventure for about four hours.

I had a TENS machine which I put on at a low level at first. About 6.00am I woke my other half up as the contractions were getting much more regular and lasting longer. I got into the bath which felt nice for a while. By 7.30am the contractions seemed to be gaining intensity and the TENS machine was up at full whack.

I phoned the hospital; they told me that for my first birth it would be a long time before I should think of coming in. Half an hour later I told Andy that I wanted to go to the hospital.

The midwife greeted me and told me it was too early but they would examine me - but I was probably better at home, until she examined me and discovered I was fully dilated and ready to push!

> I had a little gas and air which was great and then I went into the birthing pool which I found to be really great but after a while my contractions were not moving the baby down fast enough, a side effect of being a bit too relaxed.
>
> They got me out of the pool but the action of standing up was enough to make all the difference and within ten minutes Olivia was born – where I learnt she had her hand up on her head – this explained why I found the last stage of pushing so hard.
>
> I was so elated and relieved after she was born. The pressure of carrying the baby went immediately and was such a nice feeling. I could not believe how perfect she was."

Gas and air (Entonox)

A mixture of oxygen and nitrous oxide gas. Gas and air won't remove all the pain but it can help to reduce it and make it more bearable. Many women like it because it's easy to use and they can control it themselves. A lot of women find it really useful when combined with the labour breath. Some women find it makes them feel nauseous and find they can't get the technique correct. As with anything, try it and see if it works for you.

Rachel on the birth of Louie

> "I was living in central London and had been travelling over the last six years or so as, well as working.
>
> I had only met Will seven months before I got pregnant, but it was planned – although it still took me

by surprise. I moved to Kent to Will's house when I was about 12 weeks pregnant. That was a huge change as I had lived alone (mostly) for 13 years in London being very single minded... Suddenly I was now living in rural Kent and didn't know anyone which was quite hard in hindsight.

Even though it was a new relationship, Will was brilliant. In fact everyone was so thrilled (I think they thought at 39 it would never happen for me). Because of my age I did worry there would be complications. I was also fearful of the actual delivery and of making a good job of being a mum.

Louie was 11 days late. On the Thursday I was very uncomfortable and went for a walk with Will. I was going so slowly and it was so cold we gave up after about 100 metres and I went home in tears.

I had cramping and had my usual bath which stopped them. I expected to wake up in the morning with nothing happening (I was booked in for an induction on the Sunday which I was absolutely dreading).

At 4.30am I woke up with a sharp pain in my tummy and went to the loo and had a "show". I woke Will up at 5.00am who insisted on calling the hospital. They advised paracetamol and to call back at 8.30am. Within 20 minutes I was having contractions every two minutes so we rang again and I was told to go in.

We arrived about 6.00am and after about 20 minutes I was examined as I was having really painful contractions and I never got off the bed again! Louie was distressed and I had various things like a lead to measure his heart beat attached to his head (gross and really painful). I then needed to push but each contraction slowed his heart rate down really.

Another doctor took over and said one more push or it would need to be a section. I remember thinking "I don't mind, whatever," and then "NO I won't be able to drive!" I had an episiotomy and ventouse, on just gas and air. Louie was out in four pushes at 9.45am, so just over five hours after I woke up.

He needed two nights in special care as he aspirated his poo and was a poorly wee thing.

Labour wasn't too bad as it was so quick. I'm not sure I would have said that if it was hours of contractions.

After Louie was born I was just stunned. He was taken to special care after a really quick cuddle and we had to wait for quite a long time to see him. I kept asking for a shower and was told to rest. I then asked to go home, much to the midwife's amusement. She asked if I wanted to stay to see my baby, "Oh yes!" I said kind of remembering I had just had one! Where was my head?"

Injections

Pethidine or diamorphine can be injected into the muscle of your thigh or buttock and can help you to relax which can lessen the pain. It takes about 20 minutes to work and the effects last between two and four hours. A lot of women can feel quite sick when they have pethidine and it's not the most effective pain killer but if you start to feel over-anxious it may be worth a try.

Michelle had pethidine when she gave birth to Monty

"I had pethidine when I gave birth to my little boy Monty. I'd planned to have him at a birthing centre but the risk level increased while I was in labour. Things weren't progressing as quickly as they should have so the midwives said I had to go to the hospital –which was an ambulance ride away.

I was told the pethidine would stop me panicking, allow labour to carry on progressing and it would mean I'd have a fairly comfortable journey whilst being strapped to a trolley! It wasn't what I'd wanted in an ideal world but it worked a treat and the end result was that Monty and I were safe and I was able to have a normal delivery once we got to the hospital. Monty was a little sleepy afterwards but it had no adverse effect on either of us in the long run."

Epidural anaesthesia

This is a type of local anaesthetic that numbs the nerves that carry the pain from the birth canal to the brain. For most women, an epidural gives complete pain relief. It can be helpful for women who are having a long and/or particularly painful labour, or who are becoming distressed. An anaesthetist is the only person who can give an epidural, so it won't be available if you give birth at home or at most birth centres. If you're needle phobic an epidural may not be the best option for you either as it is rather big.

Another thing to note is when you have an epidural you're more likely to have intervention and there's no chance of an active labour.

Tania on the birth of Saskia Grace

"Saskia arrived on her due date. I had my first contraction about 8.30am, went to the toilet and had a show. I called my friend Helen who collected my son Kelly and took him to school for me.

My husband Dan doesn't drive so we got a cab to the Harrogate District Hospital about two miles away. I was willing the cab driver to hurry up as I didn't want him to know I was in labour.

I was already 4cm dilated when they examined me, but my waters had not broken so they did that for me. Everything was so calm and I decided to have an epidural, which I hadn't had with my first baby Kelly - and sat back to watch This Morning, I clearly remember they had some of the Bond Villains on and the man Jaws with the metal teeth.

Suddenly it was time to push; I couldn't feel a thing which was amazing. After a few pushes Saskia Grace arrived. She weighed 8lb 14oz and was beautiful.

It was a very overwhelming time, and I remember sobbing for ages afterwards. It was a new beginning for my husband Dan and me."

Here we talk to Hypnotherapist Paula Teakle about how hypnosis for birth can help during labour

"Hypnobirthing simply means using hypnosis to stay relaxed and calm during labour and birth. There are various methods but key to each one is that the mother learns and practices self-hypnosis techniques.

Women from many cultures have been tapping into the benefits of self-hypnosis and the natural ability to birth their baby for centuries but unfortunately, in the western world, childbirth has become more of a medical procedure.

Twenty years ago an American midwife named Marie Mongan developed a method called 'HypnoBirthing, the Mongan Method' (which is now a registered trademark), as a course of classes to educate parents to be to find a more gentle and natural way to bring their child into the world. These classes are taught to couples in group settings and they are designed to educate each couple on all aspects of the birth. They cover the process of birth through each stage, including breathing techniques, positioning for labour and birth, massage techniques for the birth partner to use during labour, as well as scripts for the birth partner to use and self hypnosis techniques for labour and birth.

Such self hypnosis techniques can also be learnt from a qualified Hypnotherapist, but this is not usually in a group antenatal class typesetting and, unless otherwise requested, does not usually involve the father of the baby.

When I see a client for hypnosis-for-birth session I see them on a one to one basis for the first appointment which takes place when the woman is about 32 weeks pregnant. This initial consultation is a chance for us to get to know each other and decide if we are happy to work together. A medical background is taken and then we discuss any particular issues the client may have. For example some clients have had a previous traumatic birthing experience or they may have a hospital or needle phobia.

The benefits of hypnosis for birth would be explained fully and only once the client has had a chance to ask any questions she may have, and is happy to proceed, the first hypnotic induction would take place.

Once my client is in a deeply relaxed state positive suggestions are made to help her create a 'special place' deep within her mind. A post-hypnotic suggestion is made to create an 'anchor' for the special place which can be used by the client when practicing self hypnosis at home and during the labour and birth.

In the second session breathing techniques are introduced and an exercise is done under hypnosis to release any fears and concerns.

In the third and final session pain management techniques are introduced and all previous suggestions are re-embedded. In between sessions it is important that the client practices at home using the free CDs that are supplied.

All hypnosis is self hypnosis and the hypnotherapist merely guides the client into what is a very natural and deeply relaxed state. As the body relaxes so too the mind can relax and the brain wave patterns will change.

The term for the electrical activity created in the brain when fully conscious and aware is Beta waves. As we start to relax these change to Alpha waves, then Theta waves and finally the Delta wave levels are what we experience whilst we are asleep. We all pass through these brain wave levels every time we fall asleep and every time we wake up. During the Alpha and Theta wave levels the subconscious mind is open and receptive to beneficial suggestions.

Research has shown that pain largely occurs in the presence of fear and tension. The body naturally produces and releases pain killing hormones that increase throughout labour. However when experiencing fear the body releases adrenalin which negates the effects of the pain killing endorphins.

The main benefit of hypnosis for birth is that you learn how to use your breathing to relax deeply and remain calm and in control.

Positive visualisations help to focus the mind and create a more positive expectation. Also, remaining calm and controlling your breathing conserves your energy making a long labour easier to cope with and recover from, as well as ensuring that the baby receives a good supply of oxygen throughout labour.

As long as you give your consent you can be hypnotised. We are all different and we all react to hypnosis in our own unique way. Some people are more receptive to the suggestions made and will have a more profound experience. Some women even experience a 'pain free' labour and delivery. Most women will still experience the pressure of the contractions but feel that they are comfortable and in control.

In labour you tap into the skills you've learnt. But you are not in a deep trance throughout. You use the rapid induction or 'anchor', as mentioned earlier, to slip in and out of hypnosis for each contraction. In between contractions you are able to talk and move about normally. As the contractions (or as they are referred to in hypnosis 'pressure surges') increase and get closer together, the trance level will deepen and the short time in between each one will be periods of deep breathing and rest.

You will usually have three sessions.

Self hypnosis techniques can be used alongside conventional methods of pain relief very successfully, especially TENS machines, gas and air and water birthing, so there are a variety of options throughout the labour.

As the mum-to-be feels calm she can think clearly and rationally and feel confident in her choices and decisions. Other benefits of using self hypnosis during labour and birth can be a shorter labour, reduced need for intervention, shorter recovery period, a calmer baby and reduced likelihood of post natal depression.

As home delivery becomes more common place, many women are using self hypnosis techniques to help them to feel calm and relaxed, something which is much easier to achieve in your home environment. I have also helped clients with concerns regarding conception as well as easing morning sickness symptoms.

On a personal level, I have had four children (one via forceps delivery, one via caesarean section and the last two naturally using self hypnosis). Having such a positive experience as a result of using self hypnosis I felt inspired to help other women feel empowered to have a better birthing experience, which is why I trained to become a hypnotherapist.

Not all women want to involve their partner in the hypnotic experience for a variety of reasons, many already have an in depth knowledge of labour and birth or have already attended antenatal classes and just want to focus on the self hypnosis techniques."

© **Paula Teakle Genesis Hypnotherapy 2011**

Louise's story

"I had some hypnosis-for-birth sessions and they were simply brilliant. I was a bit sceptical beforehand but I can honestly say it helped me so much. When I was in labour I just knew what to do – it all felt very instinctive. I was so relaxed and confident and my husband couldn't believe it. My baby was very chilled too and slept really well right from the beginning which is apparently common with hypnosis."

Too Posh To Push

Are some women so scared to have a baby naturally that they opt to have major surgery instead of a vaginal delivery?

Caesarean rates have more than doubled since the 1980's yet in the largest survey of recent years, carried out in 2008. It confirmed most caesareans were carried out for medical reasons.

The study published in the British Medical Journal looked at more than 620,000 single baby births in England in 2008 at 146 NHS Trusts. 147,726 were delivered by caesarean. Medical reasons were the most common. Nine out of every ten pregnancies with a breech baby resulted in a caesarean. 71% of women who had previously had a section chose to have their baby by caesarean again. There wasn't any evidence that low-risk women were being given caesareans. The rates varied widely between hospital trusts, with 14.9% at the lowest and 32.1% at the highest. They concluded the reason for this was probably the different points at which doctors decided problems in labour were severe enough to merit a caesarean.

However, things are changing. In 2011, the National Institute for Health and Clinical Excellence (NICE) said women could opt to have a section, medical need or not. A survey carried out by babychild.org.uk in the same year revealed that 51% of mothers would choose a caesarean-section over a natural birth if they had the option. Just over a third of the women surveyed claimed that the 'pain of natural birth' was the main reason behind their preference for a section, whilst 26% said they would feel 'less-stressed' knowing they were going to have a planned section. A further 18% thought that a section minimised the risk of complications and under a tenth said that they had had a bad experience when giving birth naturally before.

Cost Issues

Although women shouldn't have to worry about the cost of childbirth it is interesting how much more a section can cost.

At the end of 2011, NHS North Yorkshire and York have spoken about the costs of a section over a natural delivery. The trust said a caesarean delivery for a woman aged 19 or over costs £2,539 and for a natural birth it is £1,324. According to that one Trust, 114 women in North Yorkshire had sections for non-medical reasons during the 2010-11 financial year. If they had a natural birth it would have saved the trust £155,610.

Critics say allowing women 'too posh to push' to choose a caesarean wastes million of pounds of taxpayers' money every year.

The NCT puts the cost of a caesarean birth at £760 more than a normal delivery. They state a mere one per cent rise in the annual rate in the UK means an expenditure of £5 million that could be better spent on improving maternity care for all new mothers.

Caesarean sections are now the most commonly performed operation on women in the UK with 100,000 such operations being carried out every year. Some say that is far too many – and if the policy change does go ahead as recommended this rate will rocket.

For women, the benefits of a normal birth include improvements in morbidity rates and a quicker return home to their families. The reduction in the level of unnecessary interventions also results in a reduction of unnecessary complications. Women with spontaneous vaginal deliveries spend on average one day in hospital after delivery, women with instrumental deliveries one or two days and caesarean deliveries is three to four days (Hospital Episodes Statistics; 2004).

Increasingly celebrities are having their babies by caesarean with rumours being rife that they want to have their baby to fit their schedule. They don't want to carry the baby for too long as the most weight-gain is towards the end of the pregnancy, so they'd rather get the baby out sooner rather than later! Whether this is true or not it's apparent that what happens to famous people has an impact on the masses.

So are there any side-effects for the babies?

When you have a planned section it can be quite traumatic for the little one. Think about it – the baby is fast asleep in amniotic fluid and then is suddenly woken abruptly and torn from the place it has called home for the last nine months without any notice at all.

Babies born by section are at higher risk of developing 'transient tachypnea' which is abnormally fast breathing during the first few days after birth. Recent research also shows that babies born by planned section are more likely to become obese than those born naturally. According to doctors and scientists from Imperial College London, it's possible that the process of natural labour and passing through the birth canal enables infants to metabolise fats properly.

I would say to think very carefully about **choosing** to have a section over a normal delivery.

For many mothers the recovery period after a section is the hardest part but of course many women do have sections and the outcome is still a positive one. Here are two mums' stories:

> "I've had two children by caesarean. They both ended up being delivered by emergency section and although I would have much rather had a normal delivery I don't beat myself up about it. As soon as I laid eyes on both of my children the birth was forgotten and the most important thing was that I had beautiful, healthy children. I've resigned myself to the fact that if I have another child it will be a section and I'm not going to fight that. It is obviously the best thing for me." **Amelia**

> "I've had three sections and at each one I was so impressed with the people who were looking after me. At every stage I felt in control and that my wishes were taken into consideration." **Paula**

The reasons for a Caesarean section

There are two types of caesarean, elective and emergency. An elective section is planned before the big day and an emergency will happen once you've already gone into labour.

You may be advised to have an elective section for the following reasons:

- You have pre-eclampsia which is where your blood pressure is too high. This can have serious side effects for both mother and baby
- You have a previous medical condition that means delivery would be detrimental to you or your unborn child
- You are expecting triplets, quads or more
- You have a low lying placenta (placenta praevia)
- Your baby is transverse (lying across your tummy and can't be moved)
- Your baby is too big to be able to go through your pelvis.

Other reasons

- **Breech babies**

3-4% of babies will be breech at full term – this means the baby's head stays uppermost in the uterus with his bottom or feet positioned to come out first. Although it is possible for a breech baby to be born naturally a woman with a 'breech baby' is usually offered a section. The best thing if your baby is in breech is to see if you can encourage the baby to turn naturally.

The following may help a breech baby to turn:

- Walking for 20 minutes a day may help;
- Cat pose (hands and knees) is fantastic. You can also try rocking your hips forwards and backwards. These movements are soothing for the baby and can help if you have a stiff back or hips. Years ago our mothers would have been told to wash the floors – which was nothing to do with hygienic floors – rather being in a good position;
- Any position where you've got your hips higher than your elbows should encourage your baby to get into a vertex position so supported elbows and knees is a good one to try. From hands and knees drop your elbows down so your bottom is in the air – not very elegant I know!
- If all else fails... Try using a plank of wood. Some midwives will recommend getting a piece of wood and placing it so one end rests on a chair and the other on the floor and then lying on it – with your head at the floor end. Make sure that whatever wood you use can support you correctly and it's probably an idea to have someone nearby. Stay like this for about 20 minutes;
- Another technique to try is lying on the floor with two pillows beneath your back so that your hips are higher than your shoulders. You can also try putting your legs up the wall – but make sure you feel okay when you're lying on your back:
- From 34 weeks plus regularly adopt upright leaning-forwards positions as this will tilt the pelvis forward giving your baby more room to move. Baddha Konasana (feet together, knees apart) is a good one to try;

- Some women swear by swimming. As with anything it's worth giving it a go. If nothing else, being in the water is wonderfully soothing for a mum-to-be;
- Sit on your birthing ball as often as possible and circle or rock your hips;
- Look at the website www.spinningbabies.com for more ideas of encouraging a breech baby to turn. Beware. Some of the tips are rather hardcore!

If your baby still hasn't turned your obstetrician or midwife may discuss ways of turning the baby in the womb. This is called an external cephalic version (ECV).

Most babies are breech for no obvious reason. Premature babies are often breech and in about 40% of twin pregnancies, one baby is in the breech position.

There are a lot of different opinions about why some babies go into the breech position. Some say it is due to bad posture, particularly slouching when sitting down. Many midwives state that if a woman has 'squishy' sofas at home her baby is more likely to be in the breech position due to constantly slumping back when sitting.

Other possible conditions that make it difficult for the baby to settle head down include:

- A uterus that has a divider, or a septum running down the middle
- A tumour of fibroid low in the pelvis
- Placenta praevia
- Too much or too little amniotic fluid.

Results of an international trial of over 2000 women around the world who gave birth to babies in breech positions were published in 2000. The study concluded that it is best for a breech baby to be born by a caesarean section, as the risk to the baby was higher with a vaginal birth. However, the trial methodology has been criticised. The balance of benefits and risks is uncertain, particularly for women who may have another pregnancy. There are for example more obstetric complications following surgery, and a small increased risk of reduced fertility and stillbirth.

Mothers who plan to have a vaginal breech will need to make sure they receive care from a midwife experienced in natural breech births.

The main fears surrounding vaginal breech delivery are birth trauma and asphyxia. If the baby is small or premature there is a danger that the baby's body may deliver easily leaving the head trapped behind an incompletely dilated cervix or an inadequate pelvis.

As the rate of caesarean delivery of breech babies rises, fewer and fewer midwives and doctors are learning the skills of vaginal breech delivery. Although in theory breech babies are not necessarily benefiting from caesarean delivery, they may well be doing so in practice, because the skills of vaginal breech delivery are being lost.

Another fear associated with vaginal breech birth is cord prolapse. Since the baby's bottom or legs do not fit the pelvis as closely as the head there is more chance that the cord may slip through. However, for the same reasons the pressure on the cord may not be as great, therefore a cord prolapse with a breech may not be the immediately life-threatening event that it is with a head down baby because the foetal legs may shield the prolapsed cord from compression.

There is a school of thought that the only way you can have a breech baby vaginally is lying flat on your back with your feet in stirrups.

However, Michael Odent's natural protocol for breech birth involves no intervention whatsoever in the first stage of labour. In his book 'Birth Reborn' he says, "Insist on the supported squatting position for delivery, since it is the most mechanically efficient. It reduces the likelihood of the baby having to be pulled out, and is the best way to minimise the delay between the delivery of the baby's umbilicus and the baby's head... I would never risk a breech delivery with the mother in a dorsal or semi-seated position."

The best advice if your baby is breech is to talk through your options with your midwife and doctor – and just remember that breech doesn't necessarily mean a section. However, don't be disappointed if the advice is to have one– but make sure that they fully explain their reasons. A section can still be a positive experience – if you're prepared for it and feel in control.

> *"I was overjoyed when I first became pregnant as I was desperate to have children. I always wanted to have a natural birth but that decision was taken away with my first child because he was in a breech position with the cord around his neck - and I had to have a section. I was initially devastated. However when the baby arrived safely and the consultant told me that the cord was very short and wrapped so tightly round the baby's neck I would not have been able to deliver naturally I realised that it doesn't matter how babies comes into the world as long as they do so safely. With my second child I was disappointed that I couldn't deliver naturally but was more*

prepared for the section. I've now had three sections and each one of them has been great, and I've resigned myself that I probably won't ever have a normal labour now." **Paula**

- **Twins**

While having twins does increase the risk of you having a caesarean, fewer than half of twins are born this way.

The position of the babies plays a big part in delivering twins. About 40% of twins are both head down (vertex) at term, another approximately 30% see the first baby vertex and the second breech. Both of these positions are acceptable to consider a vaginal birth.

Over 50% of twins will be born vaginally. Whether this option is the right one for you and your babies is a discussion that should take place with your doctor or midwife. The good news is that even though you have two babies - you only have to labour once, although you do have to push twice. However twins are usually smaller, meaning that their heads are likely to be smaller too.

Sometimes, the second twin simply comes down head first like the first twin. If this is the case it is handled in exactly the same manner and is the best outcome with twins. If the second twin is breech, your practitioner may decide to allow the baby to deliver breech or they may turn the baby externally or internally. On some occasions they may do something called a breech extraction (pulling baby out by the feet).

If you are to give birth by caesarean prior to your due date, the date will most likely be set between 37-40 weeks.

Twin pregnancies can have different complications from the beginning and it's important you're well informed about labour and the possible complications. However you don't HAVE to have a section so make sure any choice you make is based on facts and not because you feel pressured into doing something you don't want to do.

> *"Do I have to have a section if I'm having twins – no and double no!"* **Emma Mahony, author of the book Double Trouble who had her twins normally with an independent midwife**

Sally talks about the birth of her twins

> *"I'd already delivered two children naturally so when I found out I was expecting twins my first thought was I wanted another natural delivery. I wanted to feel myself having my babies. The hospital was very supportive and although the labour was slightly more 'medical' than it had been with my other two children it was still fantastic.*
>
> *I delivered my daughter Sadie no problems at all – it literally took two pushes. She was head down which made it easier. My son Rupert was lying across me and they didn't know if I'd be able to deliver him normally or if they'd have to pull him out of me. However, in the event he flipped into the head down position and was delivered normally too. I was very proud of myself as just had gas and air. Not having a section meant I recovered really quickly."*

Here Michelle shares her experiences of having her twins

"My life was very hectic when I discovered I was pregnant with twins; my mum and dad had split up and my dad had been diagnosed with brain cancer. I had also just started a new job nannying for twin girls.

The baby was planned and I was lucky enough to fall pregnant very quickly, we weren't expecting to have twins though!

We joined the NCT and went along to birth preparation classes. I bought lots of books and joined lots of pregnancy websites. I knew I was going to have a section as I was having identical twins who were sharing the same placenta.

I was worried about the section and having the spinal block – and it not working properly and then having to be knocked out instead. I was adamant I wanted to be awake and be the first person to hold my babies.

Because I was having identical twins there were quite a lot of extra risks and worries throughout the pregnancy. We went for scans every two weeks to check they were both growing at the same rate. I was also worried about going into labour early and if they would go to special care and if they would be okay.

Just after my husband Dave was leaving for work on Thursday morning I had a show. I was scared for the boys as the consultant didn't want me to go into labour naturally as there were risks to the boys. I phoned Dave and he came back and rang the hospital. They said it was fine and not to worry – but I *couldn't help worrying, especially when I had another show. We rang the hospital and they said we could go in.*

After they listened to the boys' heart beats and gave me an internal, they sent me home, and said to come back in the morning for the planned section. I spent the afternoon at the hairdressers having my hair cut and coloured. I wanted to have nice hair as I knew I probably wouldn't have time to do it again for a while!

That night at 9pm my waters broke and I was scared. I was prepared for Friday not Thursday! I couldn't stop shaking!

We phoned the hospital and rushed in. We saw the consultant who said they would monitor the babies but as long as I didn't have contractions we would have a section the next day as planned. I felt a little bit better for five minutes, but then the contractions came. I only had them for about 30 minutes but the pain was awful.

Suddenly there were loads of people in the room giving me drugs and getting me ready for theatre. It was very scary but the staff were amazing and tried to put me at ease. Even though it was an emergency section the surgeon took the time to read my birth plan and even let us play music. The spinal block was amazing and I couldn't feel anything. The whole operation was amazing and suddenly they held Zachary up to me. Dave went to see him then Ashton came out.

> They were both perfect and given straight to me. I was so relieved that they didn't have to go to special care. I felt overwhelmed with love for my gorgeous tiny boys."

Previous sections

If you've already had one section it is usual to be offered another. If there has been a very small amount of time between the pregnancies it may be more sensible to consider a section as the scar won't have had time to heal and is more likely to rupture.

However, most women are capable of having a VBAC (Vaginal birth after caesarean). It's a matter to be discussed with your midwife and consultant.

Having a VBAC may mean that you'll be checked more regularly. You'll be offered continuous foetal monitoring and it's up to you to choose how closely you're monitored. See if you can still be active or not.

There is a risk that the scar from your previous caesarean could rupture which is call a uterine rupture. This happens to about one in 200 women. If the baby's heart rate doesn't sound right, it could be an early sign there is a problem with the old scar – hence the need for regular monitoring.

Louise on the birth of her second child Hector

> "My husband James and I arrived at the hospital for an elective section and waited in my cubicle for a couple of hours, reading magazines and chatting as if I was not about to give birth.

Then my slot came and we both got changed into the charming blue gowns for theatre. The team were marvellous; I had a fantastic anaesthetist and a very efficient surgeon who made me feel quite confident. I was asked if I wanted some music and thought why not, but then found the soundtrack was Old MacDonald so we ended up in silence, rather like the scientologists the team had operated on before me!

The very surreal nature of a planned birth was made even more comic by a shooting friend of James' popping his head round the door to say hello just before things got started. He was a surgeon not tourist!

At the moment of birth, I felt very excited, a little queasy, numb in lower body but very alive mentally and hugely thankful to the team for ensuring both Hector and my safe passage in theatre. I kept thanking everyone and waving a lot and I don't think I stopped talking for a while afterwards."

Abigail on the birth of her second daughter Lucy

"I had to have my second daughter Lucy by caesarean as I had a low lying placenta.

When I became pregnant with my third I didn't want a section again so had a VBAC and had a fantastic labour – even though I was induced. I enjoyed pushing Tabitha out and the recovery time was much better.

When I had my fourth daughter Olivia I had a home birth. Because I'd coped so well with the other labour and there was a seven year gap my midwife and consultant were supportive.

> *Olivia was born at home in 20 minutes – the midwife didn't even have time to arrive! Despite it being very quick and a bit of a shock it was an amazing experience and I'm glad I pushed for the VBAC and ultimately a home birth."*

The main advantage of a VBAC is you'll be in less discomfort after the birth and won't have to stay in hospital as long. Some women feel as though they miss out on the birthing process by having a section, so if you do achieve a natural birth you may have a sense of achievement.

Lisa speaks about having a VBAC with her third son Zach

> *"I'd recently started studying a course in NLP and was setting up my own business in energy medicine when I discovered I was expecting.*
>
> *My husband and I were over-the-moon even though there was a nine year age gap between this pregnancy and my last one.*
>
> *I hired an independent midwife, as I knew I wouldn't receive much advice from the NHS as it was my third pregnancy.*
>
> *I wanted to try if possible to have a natural birth this time round - my other children had been born by caesarean and I researched VBACs and decided I wanted to take this route.*
>
> *I did pregnancy yoga for the first time and had regular reflexology from 16 weeks. Towards the end I listened to a VBAC hypnotherapy CD.*
>
> *I worried about different things this time round; my main anxiety was losing the baby or the baby having*

something wrong with him. I think this came on, as I was that much older and you are aware of the complications age can bring. Also I have known women who have lost babies, either during pregnancy or in labour which made me more aware of how precious life is. Because I'd had two sections and was trying for a natural birth I was still a bit nervous.

I was four days overdue when I went into labour at midnight. My midwife stayed in touch with me on the phone and then came out the following morning, around 5am.

At some point in the morning I got into the birthing pool and with the help of gas and air and my yoga techniques stayed in there for quite awhile. Each time I had a contraction I tried to visualise my calm place. My midwife was very good at not interfering, and every once in a while she would check how far I had dilated and check the baby's heartbeat.

At around 1pm I got out of the pool and the labour pain intensified. I walked around to speed things up. At around 2pm my waters hadn't broken but I was about 9cm dilated so the midwife broke my waters and noticed some blood in the water.

She called an ambulance as we weren't sure if the blood was related to my previous caesareans. It had been snowing the week before, and there was still a lot of snow around. The ambulance put on its sirens to get to the hospital quicker, and this put the fear of God in my husband Robin as he was following behind!

Once I arrived at hospital, things changed; I dimmed the lights in the room because it was so bright. I also had to justify why I wanted a natural labour to the Registrar. Luckily my midwife, who came with me to hospital, spoke up for me.

I was fine and so was the baby and the bleeding had stopped. We agreed that I would carry on labouring for another hour. After an hour or so with plenty of squatting and pushing there was still no baby.

I was exhausted at this point and had a feeling that he was stuck, which was confirmed after an internal. I was taken down to theatre and given a spinal block. The senior consultant was called, as the Registrar didn't have experience of delivery a baby by forceps on someone who had had a section.

Finally at 6.35pm my healthy baby boy Zach was born with lots of pushing, the help of forceps, ventouse and a great team of midwives and one fantastic consultant!

Once the baby was born my exhaustion vanished to be replaced by love for this little being, and a total relief that all turned out well. I can remember the consultant congratulating Robin and me."

Emergency Sections

An emergency section can be very traumatic for mother and child. Suddenly everyone springs into efficient action and there can be a feeling something is very wrong. If you have to have an emergency section trust it's the best thing for you and your baby. It's important that you always try to keep the focus on your own health and that of your little one. If you're as calm and in control as you can possibly be you can make the best of a bad situation. This is where it's important that you've done your research and are aware of what is happening to you and why.

"When my partner had our first son by emergency section it was so traumatic, she was whisked away

from me and I had to wait in the corridor. I stood there all alone with tears streaming down my face thinking I was going to have to make a choice between her and my unborn child. Not knowing what was going on was terrifying." **Jason**

You may have to have an emergency section after labour has started because:

- Your baby's heartbeat changes – commonly known as baby becoming distressed
- The cervix stops dilating or dilates very slowly so that mother and baby become exhausted
- The placenta starts to come away from the wall or the uterus and there is a risk of haemorrhage (heavy bleeding)
- The baby does not move down into the pelvis, indicating that the pelvis is too small for the baby to get through.

An emergency caesarean can be a frightening situation for everybody concerned and it's made even worse if you're not sure what is involved. Make sure that you're aware exactly what will happen when you have a section and the differences between an emergency and an elective. When you're in labour try to remain as calm as possible – if you're calm and in control the chances are the baby will be too.

Amelia has had two children, both as emergency caesareans

"When I was pregnant with my son Marley, I was terrified about labour but I so wanted to be able to do it; I felt as if it would define me and make me a real mum.

I went into labour very early, 33 weeks + six days with my son but labour didn't progress as it should have which resulted in me having to have an emergency section.

I had joined the NCT and within my group I was the only one who had a section. I felt a failure and it bothered me for the first year as I didn't want to have one.

I had worried about how much it would hurt and how I would feel afterwards, but luckily I healed quickly and painlessly. The only thing I couldn't do was drive but that time passed quickly enough.

When I became pregnant the second time I desperately wanted a natural birth. This pregnancy and birth was going to be so different... I prepared well; I read loads, mentally visualised, tried yoga and hypnobirthing, but when the day came it was no different to the first time.

I panicked in the early stages and found I wasn't coping well. I failed to dilate during my first labour and was so scared it would happen again - and it did.

I made it to 9cm and ended up with an emergency section. The extremely scary circumstances of having another section left me numb with disappointment and anger. I raged at my body for letting me down again.

I had so wanted to hold my second baby straight away as that wasn't possible with my first baby Marley who had to go to intensive care because he was so early.

However I woke after Rani's birth to find myself alone without my baby again. It was awful and I was *extremely upset. In those minutes of waiting to see her I was so unhappy and just focusing on what had happened but the minute I saw her in my husband's arms those feelings melted away and as I held her for the first time, none of those wants or needs about the birth mattered.*

I wish I could say I carried on feeling that way but for the first few weeks I was not coping well with having had a section.

I think age had made it harder for my body to cope and my mind wouldn't let go of the birth. I dwelled constantly on not having had a VBAC. I couldn't rationalise it.

However, nature works its miracles. I have forgotten all about it and five months on I know I want another child and I know this will be a section and I can accept that now.

A caesarean ensures that your baby is born safely and as much as they are not a great experience the outcome is the same as a normal birth. You have a beautiful baby- healthy and safe in your arms."

Rachel on the birth of Amelia

"I had been through an amicable divorce and was single, living on my own and working in London when I met my now husband. We both wanted children, and it happened quite quickly.

When I found out I was pregnant I read every book I could get my hands on, watched loads of DVDs and went to antenatal classes where I met friends for life. We also started preparing the home and nursery.

I was so excited at the prospect of a new baby but there was a fear of the unknown. I also developed an itchy skin condition called Polymorphic Eruption in Pregnancy which wasn't very nice. I also worried about having my first child two days before turning 37!

My partner was a massive support throughout the pregnancy. I'd never held a baby before, so I worried about not knowing what to do. But it's true, your natural instinct takes over and you just get on with it!

I was frightened of not being able to cope – I think with first pregnancies there is a fear of the unknown. I loved being pregnant but the skin condition really made me want it over with quickly.

I had a section planned as low lying placenta had been detected early on in this pregnancy. I was just glad to know exactly when it would be happening.

The birth went to plan but a couple of days later the obstetrician had detected a heart murmur and a follow up appointment at The Royal Brompton Hospital in London would be required. Therefore what should have been a happy home-coming was tinged with sadness at the prospect of complications.

Fortunately six months later she had been given the all-clear and the tiny hole in her heart would heal naturally over the course of about five years!

Second time around I was told I would be able to have a normal delivery and all scans were reported as being fine but the weekend before I was due I started bleeding. I went to hospital where they listened to baby and told me it may just be 'spotting' and the start of my labour and to go home and rest.

However the weekend after (the day before my due date) I bled heavily. I went to hospital once again and *there I stayed all night monitoring my progress. By the next morning no progress had been made and I was still bleeding! By this time after a sleepless night I was fed up to say the least and wanted it all over.*

I opted for another section - at least it would be over and I would have my baby! After a nerve-wracking birth which left me feeling dizzy and sick my little girl was born. It was only after I had been admitted back to the ward that I was told I had lost so much blood due to low lying placenta again. I came very close to needing a blood transfusion and would have never been able to give birth naturally because of this as it could have proved fatal.

Thankfully a healthy baby arrived with no complications. When both my babies were born it was simply love at first sight; pure love, ecstasy and like a miracle had just happened. I was just on top of the world. I love being a mum - don't know why I didn't do it sooner!"

Independent midwife Virginia Howes from Kent Midwifery Practice has her own thoughts on babies being in distress:

Cardiotocography

"There is no doubt about the research in the case of foetal monitors. They have no place in a normal labour. It is much better for woman and baby to have the midwife listen to the heartbeat with either a listening device called a pinnards stethoscope or with a hand held sonic aid. On a recent television programme an interviewer said to a midwife "Technology and these foetal monitors have improved things dramatically haven't they?" The poor midwife did not know what to say because the truth is that foetal heart monitors have not improved anything.

However, women and society believe they will keep their baby safe during labour. These machines were introduced into women's labours without undergoing any research trials nearly 30 years ago. It was thought that they would indicate which babies were in danger during labour and save the lives of those babies. In nearly 30 years since their introduction, still birth rates remain the same. What has changed however is the caesarean section rate, which has risen to an unacceptably high level. One of the main reasons for the increase has been attributed to foetal heart monitors being used inappropriately during labour.

Trials that have been done since the introduction of these monitors have not found any benefits over other methods of listening to the baby's heart during labour.

Recently a multinational multi-professional task force, that included the Royal College of Obstetricians, agreed that babies do not suffer as a consequence of reduced oxygen in labour in the absence of other risk factors. Healthy babies have special mechanisms to help them to adapt to mild hypoxic (reduced oxygen) episodes during labour and birth.

Very often babies that have been perceived to be "in distress" have been born pink and screaming and full of health and so too babies that have been thought healthy have not been.

No two foetal heart patterns are the same in labour and in almost all cases the monitors are showing us variations of normal. Due to so many variations professionals cannot agree in their interpretations of the heart traces. It has been known for an obstetrician to be shown the same trace twice and give different interpretations on each occasion.

Further more when women are strapped to monitors their movements are restricted preventing them taking up the natural position of their choice. Restricted movement and lack of upright position can inhibit labour which potentially can lead to further intervention causing a snowball effect which at the end of the line is caesarean section.

The evidence suggests that foetal heart monitors should be reserved for high risk labours.

Do not let a machine take the place of someone who can keep you and your baby safe during labour, a caring sensitive midwife."

© 2000-2003 V Howes
Kent Midwifery Practice

Home births

If it all goes well a home birth can be a tremendous way to give birth to your baby. Being in your own house in familiar surroundings can make you feel empowered and in control - and being able to put your baby to bed in your own home is simply lovely.

If you are planning on a home birth though it's even more important that you know exactly what happens at each stage. You won't have the same pain relief options at home.

However, if you do make the decision to have a home birth be prepared for some disapproval. I know when I mentioned it there were some people who made it clear they thought I was being irresponsible and not thinking of the safety of myself – or my child's.

What I'd say to anyone in this situation is make an informed decision – be aware of the risks as well as the benefits and also think long and hard about yourself as a person. Are you the kind of woman who can't handle a bikini wax? If yes, then a home birth probably isn't the right place for you to have your baby – and you know what? That's okay.

There are plenty of women who still have a natural empowering labour in a hospital or birth unit. However, if you do decide to go for it make sure that you have supportive people around you for the birth. My birth partner made all the difference to me. She was amazing and the experience we shared that night long-ago is something that will bond us forever.

Even if you don't want to give birth at home, staying in your own four walls for as long as you can is ideal. Many women find that labour goes much better when they're relaxed at home, so do as much as you can where you're feeling in control before going to hospital.

There are a lot of professional bodies pushing for home births to become more common. At the moment around 2.4% of babies are born at home but this figure isn't as high as it was. In 2011 the figure fell again and many women are very wary of having a home birth.

If you decide you'd like to try for a home birth it is your right and there are many groups that can offer help and advice. Many midwifes are very supportive of women birthing at home so make sure you discuss your options – and if you meet with any negativity then ensure the reasons are explained fully to you.

Some women find the only way they can guarantee a positive homebirth is to hire their own independent midwife. If you're in the financial position to do so this may be ideal for you. As and when I have another baby, hiring one will be at the top of my list of things to do.

You'll see the same midwife every week in the comfort of your own home and that midwife will be on call once you're in labour. In the event you do have to go into hospital your midwife can accompany you – although she wouldn't be able to deliver your baby in a hospital environment it can be reassuring to have her there.

Independent midwives are fully-qualified and fully-regulated midwives who work on a self-employed babies outside the NHS. Many of them specialise in home birth and more complex cases such as VBACs, breech babies or twin pregnancies. Their skills are up to date and they are usually very knowledgeable and passionate about their jobs and the women they work with.

Virginia Howes is an independent midwife who has delivered hundreds of babies and has a high success rate of natural labours where the woman feels in control and happy with the outcome.

Virginia is very passionate about birth and believes that more women could have the birth they want to – if they get the right about of support. Here Virginia shares her thoughts about birth

"I have worked as a midwife for 15 years and have been working independently for 12 years and by now I must have attended over 500 births. I believe that given the correct conditions women without pre-existing medical conditions or high risk pregnancies can have a natural birth and all women should be able to experience an empowering birth whatever their individual situation.

Birth has become far too medical over the last 50 years. It has been turned from a normal life event into a scary dangerous situation from which women and babies have to be saved by doctors and it should not be like that. Of course there are amazing doctors who are necessary to help the minority of women who need them but the majority of women do not require help rather than calm, watchful support.

There are far too many unnecessary caesarean sections. Some of the reasons can be attributed to fear of litigation for doctors are only sued for NOT intervening when there has been a bad outcome so in some situations they jump in far too early for fear of what may lie ahead. So many women have unnecessary intervention and the words "failure to progress" are used. Some of those women are already 9cm dilated and may just need a bit more time and lots more support. The evidence is clear that there is no place for birth by the clock and using time as an indicator alone for intervention just incites more problems for both woman and baby.

The psychology of birth should not be underestimated as 90% is mental well being and positive attitude and if women are well prepared it will generally be ok. Yes it's hard work but women are designed for it. That is not to romanticise birth for we have to be honest and women need to be well aware of how birth can be, for it is painful and there will be at least one moment when a woman will be convinced she cannot do it. However with good care-givers and dedicated support she will overcome any negative thoughts and of course there are many things women can do to make birth easier for themselves.

The majority of babies could and should be born at home and the evidence from large studies tell us that home birth should be the default position and only a minority of women should go to hospital to have a baby such as women with medicals issues or if there are high risks (associated with the pregnancy).

We need more midwives – but more importantly we need more of the good ones who support woman's choice in full and who are dedicated to keeping birth normal. The care-givers role is vital during labour. If the wrong thing is said at a crucial time it can change everything. Women need positive people around who are there to empower them.

Babies are designed to withstand labour and we use the terms 'distressed' far too easily. I think if women were supported more and encouraged to do things normally rather than being pumped full of drugs, having their waters broken, encouraged to have epidurals and being made to lie on their backs birth would be very different.

We need to give the control of birth back to women. Women do not usually complain or become depressed about the pain of their labour after they've had a baby – but they do complain and reflect about the way they were treated; whether it's because they were ignored or their wishes were overlooked. That needs to change – the way we view birth as a society needs to change".

© 2000-2003 V Howes
Kent Midwifery Practice

Becky on the births of her two children, Isabella and Noah, both born at home

"Many ask me why I gave birth to both my children at home and my answer is always 'Why not?' It astounds me that something natural is now so badly understood. As long as I was fit and healthy, the baby had developed well and there were no concerns both my husband and I wanted to try for a home birth.

Some family members were very against this with the birth of our first daughter Isabella, but I believe the reason for this is a lack of knowledge or understanding on most people's parts.

I was happy with only having limited pain relief on offer as I wanted as natural a birth as possible. Having one midwife just for me once I was in labour and knowing that a second would attend for the final stages was reassuring. My husband liked the idea of being in a more familiar environment too.

On a cold December night at 4.00am my midwife arrived and I was 5cm dilated. Many hours went by before I was ready to push. Most of this time was spent chatting, the midwife and Roger drinking coffee and with me standing up every few minutes over a chair and toe-wiggling every time a contraction came. Isabella's heart beat was checked regularly, which was reassuring, and the whole atmosphere was as relaxed as it could be.

I distinctly remember that, despite the pain, being calm during this period and that was largely down to the support of Roger and the midwife Rachel - and the fact that I was in my lounge using my things whenever I wanted to.

The third stage took a good two hours but at 2:28pm I leaned back against my sofa and Isabella was born. Roger had a ringside seat of the whole thing which meant he was truly part of the whole experience.

I later discovered that Isabella was born back-to-back which explained why pushing her out was such an effort – but I did it!

With my second birth there was no hesitance opting again for homebirth even though I knew the baby was back to back again.

Often the advice is that when the baby is back to back it will be more painful and you will need intervention or pain-relief as delivery is long and hard. Having done it once before, they were happy to let me try and it certainly proved to not be a problem.

Luckily my baby decided to put in an appearance when my daughter Bella was at nursery. I'd told my friend I thought I was in labour and would she mind collecting her afterwards – so it was all really convenient.

I'm not sure whether it was the help of the birthing pool or Noah's eagerness to finally make an appearance but my third stage lasted less than 13 minutes.

My husband's face was unforgettable as he caught Noah and brought him up to the surface of the pool and later cut the cord. Was it more painful? Well I know no different but I coped with just a TENS machine, Entinox and my husband's support for the delivery of both my children.

The positive experience I had is due to the amazing midwife team that I had on each occasion. The support and encouragement, the checks they carry out and even when they close the door behind them and I was left with my new/growing family, we knew help was only a phone call away. Regular visits were made from the doctor as well as the midwife team and at no point did we feel on our own. Bella laughs at the fact that she watches TV on the sofa she was born on and we will certainly tell Noah about the big water pool we had in the lounge for him when he is older.

Giving birth is such a personal moment and each person's needs are different but being at home was certainly the best place for me."

Gemma on the birth of her daughter Isabelle

"Before I became pregnant I was working in London as was my husband Chris. We had a hectic life but a lot of fun.

I was never a very maternal person and my husband had been encouraging us to try for a baby for a several years, but I wasn't ready.

I have poly-cystic ovary syndrome so when we finally decided the time was right to try we both had to be realistic. We both agreed that if we could have children then great, but if we couldn't we wouldn't feel failures and we'd just make sure we continued to enjoy life.

As it happened, our little girl was conceived very quickly indeed – a surprise to us both. I was very lucky and had a very easy pregnancy.

I made sure I ate well and exercised a bit more gently than I used to. I walked and swam and during the latter weeks when I was on maternity leave attended prenatal yoga classes. I didn't really read a lot, but listened to my fantastic midwife and attended NCT antenatal classes.

Although people can tell you what life is like with a new baby, I don't think there really is much preparation that you can do for life afterwards. We stocked up the freezer with meals and made sure both grandmothers were on standby to help if we felt we needed it. We also tried to finish any little jobs on the house as we knew that when the little one made an entrance there wouldn't be time to do DIY in the early days.

I was very lucky that I didn't have any terrible lows. The only time I got sad was when the NHS midwife didn't really have time to answer my questions and I felt like I was in a factory being processed along a belt. That was when my husband found our independent midwife, Virginia Howes.

Once we'd met Virginia I felt able to make choices about birth, choices that I hadn't known existed! I got angry at the NHS as I now realise that I wasn't given all the options available. I'd been told that my first baby should be born in hospital as it's safer, but as it turns out, research shows (that providing you have a 'normal' pregnancy) it's just as safe if not slightly safer to have a first baby at home.

Once we'd decided to have an independent midwife I certainly looked forward to every visit from Virginia and felt reassured that my decisions were based on fact and I knew that she would support my choices every step of the way. Unlike many women, I wasn't scared about giving birth. I think I felt so prepared and had so much faith and trust in Virginia, I just knew things would be okay. I knew she had my best *interests at heart and would do everything in her power to make my birth experience as positive as she could.*

During the afternoon of the 20th December I started feeling very mild cramps in my tummy so called Virginia as snow was beginning to come down thick and fast. She didn't think I was in active labour yet but decided to make her way to us as we live on the top of a hill up a country lane which becomes pretty nasty in the snow.

When she got to us in the evening we had a chat over a cup of tea and she agreed that she thought things were beginning to happen but said things could take a while yet. Due to the weather, she decided to stay with us just in case and went up to bed in our spare room.

At midnight I started to have quite strong contractions, so she came downstairs to support me. Chris filled up the pool with water and I got in for the pain relief and my waters went.

We kept things really calm with low lighting, music, a log fire and the Christmas tree lights on. I remember those last few contractions whilst going through the transition phase – boy did they hurt!

I was never checked as Virginia knew from how I was behaving exactly what stage of labour I was in and she just let nature take its course.

After pushing for a little while I got out of the water as Virginia didn't feel that baby was moving as quickly as it should. After a couple more contractions and an examination it turned out that the baby's chin was up and had got stuck. Once her chin was popped down she began coming pretty quickly.

Not long afterwards our little girl was born in one go - none of this head out then body at next contraction! She came out kicking and screaming to a very emotional mummy and daddy.

We both cried our eyes out. As her head was crowning I closed my eyes and imagined myself as the baby coming out of a tunnel of darkness into the light – I just saw a crescent of light getting bigger and bigger.

We left our baby's cord pulsing whilst we held her and found out that she was a little girl then Chris cut it.

My placenta was out within a couple of minutes and Virginia massaged my uterus to get it to contract.

My amazing midwife then whizzed around and tidied everything up whilst Chris made us all tea and toast. She stayed with us for the next five hours to make sure that Isabelle was feeding well and that I was okay and then left us to it.

It was so lovely to be at home, I really can't believe I managed it without even gas and air!

A few days later when we were discussing the birth with Virginia she explained exactly what had happened when the baby's head got stuck. She said if I was in hospital they would not have left me to push for so long (two hours I later found out) as hospital policy is to allow a mother to push for one hour before intervening. If I had been in hospital I probably would have been cut and forceps or another tool used.

I am so pleased that Virginia had confidence in her skills as a midwife and mine as a mother giving birth as I had the experience I wanted in the end. I owe her a lot.

I was so lucky that at the moment of birth I felt absolutely amazing. I was of course relieved that it was all over and amazed that I had just given birth. I couldn't believe that I'd done it. I was so emotional and felt drained and weak, but absolutely elated."

Catherine on the birth of her daughter Lola

"I had a really positive home birth because I took responsibility and gathered as much information about labour and what my body would have to do during birth. I did a lot of research and went to aqua aerobics and pregnancy yoga. I also paid for antenatal sessions and bought a hypnobirthing CD. For me a turning point was watching a birthing programme called Cherry Has a Baby. It looked so peaceful - I knew that was the way I wanted my baby to be born. I read up about water and home births and hired a heated pool. I discovered having a baby in water makes it much less painful and I was determined to do it that way in the comfort of my own home. I wouldn't talk to anyone who said it was going to be horrific.

My waters went at 6.30pm on January 30th. I rang the hospital to let them know and they said to contact them again once my contractions were regular and the community midwife would come. I remained active and sat on my birthing ball.

By 10.30 pm I thought ouch, and got into the pool. I knew it was important not to get in too early as the water can slow things down. By this time it wasn't the most comfortable thing but it didn't hurt. I breathed through it all which helped.

When the contractions felt strong I reminded myself that every one took me closer to meeting my baby. By 12.10 am my contractions were three minutes apart.

The midwife arrived at 12.30 am and Lola arrived at 1.03 am.

The birth was exactly the way I wanted it to be. Throughout my labour we listened to Magic Radio and all the songs were those we played on our wedding day. For me understanding what was happening at every stage is what made it so wonderful. The information is there but you have to find it. If I was to have another child, I wouldn't change a thing."

Alex on the birth of Martha

"At about 4am I was woken up by tightening sensations. I was ten days over the official, slightly dubious, due date and didn't want to get excited too soon that this would be 'it'. We were booked for a home birth and had been working really hard to make this birth as positive an experience as possible and knew that we were on the verge of losing the privilege of having this, our second birth, at home. But they did feel different – over the top of my bump as well as underneath. It seemed like a good sign…

Reluctantly, I asked my husband Mike if he could work from home again. I didn't really want him to miss another day at the office for the sake of another false alarm, but by the morning the tightenings were still happening and I was really hoping that this time they would keep going. It was our daughter Ella's first day back at nursery after half term and I'd had a feeling that things weren't going to happen until she was back and I could focus on the job that needed doing.

I had an appointment with the midwife booked for that afternoon so decided to carry on as normal, get some things done and ask her opinion on these tightening sensations when I saw her. So I headed into town to take the dog to the groomers, do a food shop and fill up the car.

By the time I dropped off the dog, the tightenings were still coming. The groomer, a lovely guy with five children of his own, was quite calm about this and assured me that should my waters break in Sainsbury's he would look after Rosie and bring her home for me.

It was during the food shop that I began to think that these sensations might go the distance. I also started to get a measure of how frequently they were coming by how many aisles I'd been down since the last one. As time went on, the gaps between only allowed me to get from one end of an aisle to the other. Having the trolley to lean on was helpful and I did find myself becoming more engrossed in whatever happened to be on the shelf next to me. Still, no one else in the shop would have noticed and between these moments I felt normal and carried on with the shopping.

By the time I left the shop I was daring to hope that this would be it. It was about 10.45am so I loaded the shopping into the car (slowly!) and got in to wait for the call to collect Rosie. At this point I decided to call Mike and suggest that, if he had time, he might start putting the plastic sheeting down in the room we were going to use. As I sat in the car the tightenings were becoming more pronounced and sitting down through them was less comfortable than walking around had been. I sat and talked to the baby to tell her that she was doing so well and that today would be a really good day to be born. 'Keep going' I told her.

I decided to keep moving, so went to the groomer's to see if Rosie was ready. She was still being preened so I walked slowly around the shop. Two tightenings later I decided more walking was what I needed so headed off around the block. At the end of the first tightening that made me want to stop and lean on something, the groomer appeared with Rosie. I took her to the car and headed home. I would have gone straight there but there was no queue at the forecourt so nipped in to fill up the car. I hadn't been paying serious attention to how frequent these sensations were, but when I had one filling up the car, one paying for it and one half an mile down the road it dawned on me that they couldn't be too far apart and I really should be getting home.

Once home I called the delivery suite to ask them to get my midwife to call me. I felt a bit of a fraud as I *was perfectly calm and my voice was normal. It still felt like the right thing to do. While I waited, Mike made me some soup and I ate it bouncing gently on the birthing ball and watching television. I was determined that I was not going to go into this birth hungry and risk running out of energy as had happened last time.*

My midwife, Ruth, rang shortly before 1pm and we had a chat about what was going on. We went over the length of my previous labour (about a day and a half) and Ruth advised me that this one would probably be quicker but that it didn't sound as though there was a rush at the moment. Someone would be out to me this afternoon but to call if it felt as though things were speeding up.

The tightenings were getting more intense and Mike put the TENS machine on me. It was a lovely feeling – a bit like lying on a foot spa! I was using the breathing I'd learnt through hypnobirthing to work with each tightening by this time. I'd lean forward onto something, breathe in really slowly, visualizing my uterus expanding upwards and outwards to make each wave do as much work as possible to dilate my cervix. Between each one I was moving around as normal and indulging in some serious nesting. It was suddenly very important to get Ella's room and the bathroom cleaned. Mike was finishing getting the birthing room ready, taping the plastic sheet to the skirting, taping an old duvet cover on top of it, gathering chairs and old sofa cushions to lean on and covering the sofa bed. He also covered the landing with plastic to give a covered route to the bathroom!

The room looked and felt lovely – a calm blue colour, pictures to remind me of key visualisations, flowers and calm music. I remember the sun catching the crystal in the window and filling the room with rainbows and thinking there was nowhere else I'd rather be to give birth to this baby. We'd worked hard together to prepare for this birth and now I was sure it was going to happen soon and I was so grateful to feel excited rather than fearful.

Still, there was no time to just sit and stare. The cleaning wouldn't do itself and I was getting frustrated that I wasn't able to get as much done between the surges! Mike began timing them, much to my annoyance. I was convinced that because they didn't feel that intense that they weren't doing much and I was preparing myself for a long time ahead. I just wanted to keep doing things to pass the time. Mike, on the other hand was becoming convinced that things were moving along much more quickly. His recording showed that each surge was lasting 45-60 seconds and that they were coming roughly every two and a half minutes. My perception was way off. I thought they were only lasting 10 seconds and was just annoyed that they were interrupting my cleaning! At around 2pm I began to feel a sense of urgency that we stop cleaning and preparing and get into the birthing room, put on my hypnobirthing CD and drop into a state of calm. Mike had a few phone calls to make to arrange for Ella to be picked up from nursery and looked after overnight if necessary. Unbeknownst to me, at about 2.30pm he also put in a call to the midwife. He was beginning to think he might have to deliver our second child himself as I had apparently begun to go into 'the zone'.

I had just got changed into an old shirt and put on the CD and was having the first feelings of self-doubt. In retrospect, I was clearly at transition; although I was still convinced I needed to prepare myself mentally for a good few hours yet. The surges were becoming stronger and I needed to be on my hands and knees rocking forwards and backwards to make them easier. My breaths were becoming louder as I had to let out the energy of each surge. There was no doubt in my mind now that these were actually doing something! And then I felt an urge to push at the end of one surge… even then I was still convinced I must still have a long way to go.

A few minutes later, at 2.55pm one of the community midwives, Debbie, arrived. She spoke to Mike on the way upstairs and came in to see me. I wasn't really able to speak to her other than to say hello before concentrating on the next surge. She gave Mike her phone and asked him to call my midwife and tell her to come now, as she didn't have as much time as she thought she had. Maybe I was closer than I thought.

She came into our room to see me and couldn't have been more wonderful. She eased into the calm atmosphere, speaking to me quietly and apologizing for asking to examine me and listen to the baby's heartbeat. She monitored the baby for a few seconds, just long enough to get a good heartbeat, and then she examined me. To my amazement (but not Mike's!) she told me I was fully dilated and I could go with the urge to push the next time it came. I remember feeling so overwhelmed with joy and disbelief that I had finished the first stage that I cried. The thought that I was already there was so wonderful. Then those wonderful words: 'Let's get you into the position you want to be in for delivery.' Not the position that was most convenient for her, but what I felt was best for me and our baby. With help from Mike and Debbie, I got back onto my knees and rested my arms and head on a stack of old sofa cushions. She then encouraged me to do what my body wanted to do and gave me the confidence to use each surge. Mike was right there reminding me to breathe our baby down and I felt the baby join in by pushing up with her feet as her head was bearing down.

As she halfway down, my waters broke, creating a wonderful feeling of extra space. Debbie quickly monitored the heartbeat and confirmed that the baby had coped with that fine – 'She's laid back about that' she told us. Just a few minutes later I could feel her beginning to crown. I had the feeling that I just couldn't get any fuller and had a moment of doubt as to whether she could possibly get out. I felt the instinct to tense up. That was when I remembered the visualization of the opening rose that had been part of our hypnobirthing preparation. I'd found a beautiful photograph of one and had it in the room with us. Taking a calm breath and thinking of that rose, I felt myself relax and seconds later heard Debbie say that the head was out: no tearing, no cutting. I was stunned and felt a little shocked that we were now definitely at the end of this birth experience. With the *next surge our lovely daughter was born into our spare bedroom, with one lovely midwife there to catch her and the sound of my hypnobirthing CD beginning to count up from 1 to 10 to bring me back into the room, only 45 minutes after we had put it on. It was 3.20pm.*

Our little girl was quiet and calm, not crying, but Debbie reassured me she was fine. I turned over and brought her onto my chest, not really able to believe that we had done it. We had had a few names in the running but when we met her, the only one to suit her was the soft, calm sounding 'Martha'. It didn't really take any discussion to agree that this was right for her. Debbie clamped the cord and Mike cut it. Ten minutes later, my midwife, Ruth, arrived and joined us. We had opted for a natural third stage and so enjoyed a wonderfully calm half an hour with us all sat on the floor, Martha and I covered in towels. Mike brought up tea and biscuits and Martha began to feed.

Martha's suckling really encouraged the placenta to come away. With a little palpitation and a few pushes, I delivered the placenta, amazed by how the whole process is designed to work. Debbie and Ruth cleared away what little needed taking away and took some very precious photos. They then helped me to the shower whilst Mike had a wonderful cuddle with Martha.

As I came out of the shower, our friend, Sam, arrived to collect the car seat on the way to collect Ella. I called her up, her face full of concern asking how it was going. When I said she should go in to meet Martha, concern switched to shock and the exclamation 'I thought your waters had just broken!' She joined us at about 5pm, just as the midwives were preparing to leave. I felt great, Martha was happy and healthy and we were loving basking in the magical atmosphere of that afternoon.

Mike went to collect Ella from our friend, Ali's house just around the corner, where she had enjoyed having tea with her little boy, Gus. Ella came home meet her new sister after hardly any change to her day. She was unsure initially and asked to see my tummy. After commenting that it had 'burst' she seemed confident that this was indeed the baby that had been in there this morning. When she got into her pyjamas and asked if the baby could sleep with her, we knew we were okay!

With Ella in bed, Martha dressed in an outfit Ella had chosen and me also in pyjamas there was only one thing left to do – the one thing that was top of my priority list this time after my experience recovering from giving birth to Ella in hospital three years before – we ordered a pizza! Mike and I spent the evening snuggled on our sofa together enjoying every bite, cuddling our new daughter, and beginning to spread the word of her arrival."

And sometimes a baby is born at home – when that wasn't in the plan...

Taryn on the birth of Dexter

> *"My eldest son Jarrad was 28 months when my next son Dexter decided upon an accelerated entry into the world.*
>
> *It was a very different experience to the 19 hours that I had endured with my first baby.*
>
> *It had just gone midnight when I woke up with a tummy ache and decided to get out of bed and walk around the bedroom. 15 minutes later I was still uncomfortable but not in pain and thought this could be the onset of labour.*
>
> *Despite this being my second baby I referred to the manual on signs of labour and decided to call the hospital to see if I could come in just for a check-up.*
>
> *My husband called our friend to see if she could look after the eldest and within 10 minutes she arrived.*
>
> *As my husband let her in the front door I came walking down the stairs to get my shoes on. Just before I touched down on the last stair I decided I needed the bathroom and walked back to the loo….lucky I did. As I sat down my waters broke and within seconds the contractions hit me like an arctic lorry. I had gone from' mildly uncomfortable' to' someone please get this out of me **NOW**!'*
>
> *My husband came running up the stairs and I told him I was not going to the hospital I was not leaving! He called the hospital and they said they would send out a midwife and assume an unplanned home birth and recommended that "just in case" my husband should call an ambulance.*

As the 999 operator was talking to my husband I was screaming that the baby was coming, at this point I had managed to move the 10cm from the loo to bearing down my weight on the hand basin.

The 999 operator advised my husband to move me into the bedroom and off the ceramic tiled floor.

As my husband paled with the operator telling him he could talk him through the birth the midwife arrived, closely followed by a rapid response paramedic and the standard ambulance with two crew.

I now had my husband, my friend, four medical personnel and two cats in my bedroom. The midwife examined me told me we were good to go and with no pain relief and after a labour that was recorded at only 52 minutes my second son entered the world on the bed, where he had been conceived and with a room full of spectators.

By 4am the house was quiet again, and my husband and I went back to bed with our newborn in the crib.

Later that morning Jarrad came running in to our room to say good morning and having slept through the whole situation during the night, he finally met his brother."

But some people are against home births and think that as things do go wrong women should be in hospital – or at the very least a birthing centre with a hospital close by.

Here, mum of three Dr Helen Terrell shares her thoughts on birth

"I believe that it is important for mums to be able to make a truly informed decision about where they should deliver.

The problem is that a normal, healthy pregnancy does not guarantee you a low risk, complication-free birth.

I think there is no doubt that generally mums do well in any environment with the right support. They progress more slowly in hospital attached to monitors, when they are less mobile.

However, as a junior doctor, I attended many deliveries as an emergency when deliveries have not gone to plan. It is not possible to predict who will run into problems. Babies get stuck (shoulder dystocia), the cord can prolapse; they can fall out of the cervix disturbing the blood supply and babies develop bradycardia (slow heart rate).

I've attended a delivery in the past, where the baby was having a normal delivery, got stuck and a midwife had to travel with her fist up the vagina from the delivery suite to get the baby out by a caesarean section!

If not hospital, I think a birthing centre, located in a hospital with a specialist obstetric and paediatric unit would be my ideal.

In the past, I have always been an advocate of normal vaginal delivery, but my own personal experience has now completely changed my view.

I have carried all my babies breech and have been offered a section on each occasion. I had James and William both turned by ECV to enable a vaginal delivery. James was meant to be a water birth. I was pushing and was suddenly hauled out of the water because his heart rate had dropped. I was told there was no time for ventouse and James was born very flat (floppy) by forceps and episiotomy. He recovered quickly, but I have no doubt that had I been at home, or the birthing centre, the outcome would have been very different, with either a fatal outcome or at least brain damage.

By definition, you are low risk to be allowed to try a water birth...

My waters broke with William my second baby and I went into hospital. I wasn't progressing and they tried to send me home for a bit. My intuition knew that this was not right and I loitered in the park next to the hospital for a polite time before going back to delivery suite!!

They examined me and I was only 4cm. I was having strong contractions and William's heart rate was dipping, suddenly a dip did not recover and I was being raced on a trolley down the corridor for an emergency section.

Had I not been at hospital, again the outcome could have been very different. I had a miserable time post forceps delivery. I bled a lot, was bruised and was unable to sit comfortably for weeks. The anaemia kyboshed my hopes of breastfeeding. I can't say I really enjoyed the first three months and I'm sure the miserable start didn't help.

My section recovery was lots better. I was mobile in 24 hours and recovered quickly. I was in a much better state to enjoy my baby and toddler than the last time.

Third time I thought I'd have a nice controlled planned section, but then my waters broke a week early!

To any woman I would say; be realistic that there will be changes of plan and go with the flow. Trust the professionals to act in your best interests."

My top tips:

- Try to relax as much as you can
- There is NO point feeling guilty that you didn't get your perfect delivery. Few people pop them out like peas!
- Water, water and more water... getting in the birthing pool was fabulous
- Keep upright and mobile as much as you can
- Get the right midwife for your personality! (I needed a much more assertive one than the first airy fairy one!)

© 2011 Dr Helen Terrell

Some women love becoming a mum so much they have lots of children... Here we speak to Giselle Green, best-selling author and mum of six boys about motherhood and what it means to her

"I thought becoming a mother would be a whole lot easier than it was. I remember innocently (!) asking a work colleague who'd just had a baby 'what do you **do** all day?' I honestly had no idea how much time and energy it takes to look after a child.

For one thing, I thought babies slept a lot, at least at the beginning. My first-born only ever seemed to nap if I was pushing his pram or driving around in the car. The sleep-deprivation was debilitating. I remember a friend saying she 'couldn't wait' till her daughter was nine weeks old and slept through the night – none of mine seemed to do that till about the age of two. As we had six children in nine years, there were eleven years of broken sleep... I can't imagine going through that now.

I also had no idea how much I would need to slow down once the children came along. That's not a bad thing but it takes some getting used to. A little shopping trip into town that I'd do in half an hour before became a three-hour monumental task. When you have a small child in tow, then that child is the central focus of your attention – you have to squeeze the other stuff, like the shopping, in at the edges, and around their timing. Accompanying a toddler that wants to stop and examine every blade of grass along the road can seem frustrating at first, but once you learn to slow down a little and match their pace, life becomes entirely more enjoyable! Obviously that doesn't mean the child takes the reins and you never have to chivvy them along, you find a balance. Children notice things that we have forgotten how to notice, and they enjoy little things we have forgotten how to enjoy too.

There are things that you can't ever really know until you experience them for yourself – and becoming a mother is one of these things. You can't explain to someone who's never experienced 'love at first sight' that that is exactly how it is when you meet your newborn. Then again, if you listen to some of the tales of woe about the pain of childbirth, for instance, you might decide never to go there and then you'd never know that there are other very powerful factors that come into play that mitigate all that.

Maybe the main thing to remember is that – even though many of us enter parenthood pretty clueless – there's nothing about it that's going to be impossible for us to learn. Most of it we will get right first time and what we don't, we will put right in time.

And sometimes there are phases – like toilet training – that we simply have to cope with; there aren't always ways to expedite them, no matter what other people tell you.

If I was to give advice it would be don't forget to enjoy your baby! There's so much to take in when a child first comes into your life and we want things to be perfect – from making sure the place is clean enough, to knowing the right way to deal with the child when he/she's distressed.

Half the time if you let your instincts guide your actions you'll know exactly what to do.

Let yourself off the hook with regards to immediately losing the 'baby weight' too. Your baby doesn't care if you're a 'yummy mummy' – to them, it only matters that you're a happy mummy.

I've changed profoundly since becoming a mother. It's changed the way I look at things entirely. It's made me trust my instincts a lot more. I think most mums find they have a natural way of tuning into their children, a sense of being connected to them. I remember one time I was vacuuming a bedroom and my toddler was in crawling around in the next room which at the time was completely empty. Then something alerted me to danger. I switched off the vacuum cleaner and rushed in just in time to rescue him from silently choking on a tiny piece of plastic he'd found on the floor. Over time, if you allow it, that sense of connection can extend far wider than to just your own children. It's made me more empathic with other people, too.

Having trained initially as a scientist, I used to be more 'in my head,' working things out logically. Whenever I have to make a decision nowadays, I still look at the logic of things but I let my gut instincts have the final say in the matter. I've learned to trust that, and I know that's something that's opened up because of becoming a mum."

© 2012 Giselle Green

Part Three

The Reality

GIVING birth is an emotive subject and the fact is many women are frightened. Society doesn't help with the negative images and reports of labour and well-meaning friends and colleagues do little to put a pregnant woman's mind at ease and it seems unless you pay to hire an independent midwife or attend pregnancy yoga or hypnobirthing you're alone.

Midwives just don't have the time to spend with women and that's a sad fact. When I had my midwife appointments I always felt as though I was being rushed out of the door and that wasn't the Midwife's fault – I knew she had a packed clinic every time, but there wasn't any ever time to chat and talk about concerns and most mums-to-be have a few of those!

If there was more time and support for women, the number of interventions and caesarean sections would go down saving the NHS a fortune.

In 2000 an article published in the British Journal of Psychiatry described the fear of childbirth or pregnancy as a psychological disorder, when it had previously received little or no attention before. If you're particularly scared of giving birth it's even more important to find out how you can help yourself. Look into hypnobirthing or prenatal yoga and talk to women who have had positive birth experiences – they are out there. Try not to allow other people's negativity to impact on you. If it's a real issue you can discuss your fears with your midwife and doctor as you may be a suitable candidate for cognitive behavioural therapy which may be free on the NHS in extreme cases. There is lots you can do so don't spend the whole of your pregnancy worrying and being fearful, sometimes these worries can be a self-fulfilling prophecy.

In 2011 actress Tilda Swinton described giving birth as a truly murderous business. The Oscar-winner went on to say the idea that giving birth is "all really lovely" puts extra pressure on women who are struggling to cope with the shock of motherhood. Anyone who has had a baby knows how violent the process of birth is and something women need to embrace in order to accept what they're going to have to endure.

With those kinds of statements appearing in the media it's no surprise that many women are genuinely terrified.

In addition it seems that people queue up to tell you how awful their labour was which is not particularly useful.

Many women report that for the first time in their lives they are approached by strangers who feel they have the right to impart the details of their own harrowing experience of birth onto them. Why?

This is one time in your life you should be a bit rude if need be and just say to the other person that you don't want to hear their horror stories and they would do well to keep their opinion to themselves.

On the other side of the coin some women look down on women who haven't had a natural labour – and that's not right either. Smug should be kept out of giving birth and being a mum – otherwise it will only come and bite you on the bum at some point.

When supermodel Gisele Bundchen had her son Benjamin in 2009 she claimed it didn't hurt in the slightest... She said she wanted to be very aware and present during the birth and didn't want to be drugged up.

Hmmm I'm not entirely sure how useful that is for women to hear.

Of all the women I've ever spoken to about giving birth, even those who have a good labour, I've never heard anyone say there wasn't **any** pain. I think Gisele's points are valid but she sounds very judgemental and a little bit superior which isn't particularly supportive for other women. Combine that with the face of an angel and an incredible body – I can't imagine she has many female friends!

You only have to log onto any baby/mum-to-be chat room and you'll witness the swell of emotion and fear that giving birth evokes. There's a lot of judgement and negativity surrounding the choices that women make which is a pity. If society was more supportive perhaps that would all change?

Giving birth is something that most women will go through and yet there are so many negative connotations attached to it and there have been countless women who have had such a bad time in labour that the Birth Trauma Association has been set up in order to help women who have had a harrowing experience.

According to the Birth Trauma Association's latest statistic it is estimated that in the UK alone, 10,000 women a year may develop Postnatal Post Traumatic Stress Disorder (PN PTSD). As many as 200,000 women may also feel traumatised by childbirth and develop some of the symptoms of PTSD. Approximately 1/3 of women have some traumatic response to birth.

It's really sad that so many women spend their whole pregnancies worrying about what's going to happen to them in labour and dreading giving birth. Our society has somehow ingrained in the majority of women that having a baby is horrible and something to just be endured rather than enjoyed.

> *"I felt really upset when I told my work colleagues that I was planning a natural labour and was going to try hypnobirthing. They literally surrounded me and told me I'd never be able to do it and that it was so painful that the only way you could get through was with loads of drugs.*
>
> *I started to doubt the choices I'd made. After speaking to mums who had had a good labour I decided that I'd keep my opinions to myself and only share my thoughts with other like-minded women."* **Charlie**

Yes it is painful – but it is endurable and there are many, many things that you can do to make the experience a good one.

If you find you are getting worked up and agitated - stop and think about what's happening to you and to the baby when you're stressing and worrying. There has been a lot of research conducted into babies picking up on their mother's emotions when they're in-utero. Being relaxed and positive will help you both.

It's not about having an unrealistic view of labour and having a baby, like our friend Ms Bundchen. It's about preparing yourself mentally and physically for what's going to happen and focusing on the things you can do to make it as good an experience as possible. It's not all candles burning and soft music playing – although that does happen for some women. There are many, many women who have a tremendous experience in labour and you too could be one of them.

Virginia Howe's Independent Midwife RN, RM, BSc (HONS) gives her top tips:

- Take control of your birth experience
- Go to a variety of pre-natal classes, including different exercise classes
- Speak to as many women as you can with children and look for common themes between those who had a good or a bad experience
- Dismiss the scaremongering and just focus on the facts
- Remember we are put on this earth to do this – trust that your body will not let you down.

So what does the average woman think about birth and motherhood?

"Honestly. I was petrified! I had no idea what it was going to be like or how to take care of a baby, but I guess deep down I knew that my natural maternal instincts would kick in once he was born, and I was right! Like a duck to water I was!!!" **Stacy**

"I was quite ignorant about the whole thing before I fell pregnant, I just thought it was what we women are made for and therefore the whole thing should come naturally and easily." **Tannita**

"I was worried about being out of control and panicking but when it came to it I was really calm. My most resounding thought half way through, was this isn't too bad. It wasn't – but I wouldn't want to do it every day!" **Rachel**

"My thoughts about labour before I had my son were probably like most expectant mothers… magically thought out and probably a bit unrealistic. I thought it would go exactly to plan; I'd have my birthing pool set up in the living room alongside my play list and snacks.

But in the end I had to go into hospital, very reluctantly as my waters had broken but nothing had happened. However because labour ended up being very long and my baby over 10lbs being in hospital was the best thing for us." **Jo**

"I worried about the birth and also losing the weight afterwards." **Taryn**

*"I was really scared about having too much medical intervention. Both my babies were breech until 36

weeks and I was dreading being forced to have a section when I really didn't want one." **Marianne**

"I was petrified, mainly because I knew I would have to let my body take control and not my head." **Helen**

"Having been told I was going to have a section which I was prepared for I was then told I was in fact going to give birth naturally. I was so scared and unprepared – the end result was an emergency section." **Virginie**

"I was frightened of losing control and unimaginable pain that would go on forever. I also worried that labour would come on when I was out shopping and I'd have to run home." **Tamandra**

"I was afraid of the pain (quite normal I think?) And the unknown. Being a mum later in my life than I had expected I would I was also worried that as I was almost 30 I may have problems during pregnancy. Before I fell pregnant I was not convinced that I would ever be able to conceive." **Tannita**

"Will I be physically and mentally strong enough to deal with the pain and demands of childbirth?" **Rebecca**

"I didn't have any preconceptions about motherhood. I was unprepared for the unrelenting slog of broken sleep and constant things to do, nor the rewards of seeing your children learn something for the first time or the joy you can feel giving them a cuddle or listening to their little conversations!" **Helen**

"I was afraid of the birth as I'm sure all women are. None of my close friends had any children yet so I couldn't grill them on what exactly to expect, I was more afraid of the not knowing what was going to happen. I was also petrified of needing an epidural as I hate needles! Luckily I didn't need one but can now see why some women end up begging for one! And then of course there is the worry of what it could do to your 'lady bit's' and all the horror stories you hear. It's enough to send anyone into a blind panic!" **Samantha**

"I was simply terrified; I just didn't think I'd be able to cope with the pain. In the end I confronted it head on and did a course of hypnobirthing, went to pregnancy yoga and found a really good antenatal group. By the time I was nine months pregnant I was fully prepared and labour was good. Something I never would have believed possible." **Nicola**

"I spent most of the time looking at everything through rose tinted glasses. I had visions of this perfect little family that we were about to start and how great it would all be, which of course it was but I didn't think of how we would cope financially after the baby arrived. I was a bit naïve and just assumed I would go back to work part time, which I soon found out wouldn't be the case." **Samantha**

"When I discovered I was pregnant I decided I wanted all the drugs on offer but the more I learned the more I was determined I wanted a natural homebirth and I did." **Catherine**

"I assumed because I'd worked as a nanny for years I would know exactly what to do and it would be easy. I was wrong as I didn't ever factor in the bond/love/attachment that you feel for your own babies." **Michelle**

"I'd had my two elder boys by caesarean and when I became pregnant again I didn't want another section. I employed a private midwife, went to yoga every week and had reflexology. I took control of my pregnancy – something I hadn't done before. I felt as though I knew what I was doing. When I had Zach it was the experience I wanted. I had him naturally and was very proud of myself." **Lisa**

"I was petrified of pain and a tad worried about the total loss of control and dignity. However, my main concern was for a healthy baby and me." **Louise**

"All I could think about was how much it was going to hurt. I tried to block out how I was going to cope with the pain. I'd decided I would use all the drugs I could just to get me through – however, that wasn't meant to be. I went into labour three weeks early so there wasn't any time to prepare and in the end I just got on with it, and it wasn't that bad. In fact I'd go as far to say is it's the most rewarding experience of my life."
Joanne

Sometimes the reality is so very different from the expectation as Karen shares

"I had very little idea of what either entailed and so had this romantic vision of sailing peacefully and smilingly through the days with a compliant, happy baby who would be loving and want to do whatever I was doing. My baby would naturally be dressed in gorgeous clothes and have tasteful, magical toys and I would be competent and confident with my newborn embracing swimming lessons and baby massage. She and I would have wonderful easy days with a little bit of fairy dust!

As for the birth I dismissed all the nonsense about pain relief - I had endured 20 years of extremely painful periods so a spot of labour would clearly be no bother to me! I went along to the hospital visit feeling strongly that it was not relevant to me and that the people there could offer me nothing of use.

I was bemused by the nerves shown by other expectant mothers and shuddered at the cold clinical and frankly scary birthing room we were shown feeling thankful that I would not be going anywhere near it.

I had a home birth planned and did everything I could to keep myself fit and healthy. I used lots of positive affirmations and visualisations of the birth I desired. (I had a little smile at the midwife's reaction to my birthing plan - 'I'm not going down the hospital route of being pulled around and made to lie on a bed when it is obvious to anyone the most natural way to give birth is squatting - have you ever tried to poo lying on your back? I mean, let gravity help out, for goodness sake!' I believed I was bound to be different to all the other women she sees...

The reality was so different. I had a long, gruelling labour and despite my partner filling up the birthing pool that I hired for my planned home birth I didn't even put a toe in it. I had to go to hospital as things weren't progressing.

When my daughter finally made her appearance into the world it was so different to the way I'd planned it in my mind. Her shoulder got stuck and she was literally pumped out of me – it was horrific and something that troubled me for a long time afterwards.

However, I realise it was lucky I was at the hospital rather than at home – if I'd been there the outcome could have been so different. It's made me realise that there are things you can't plan to the letter and birth is certainly one example of that."

Osteopath Richard Whitworth has worked with many pregnant women and their babies and shares his thoughts surrounding birth

"I believe a lot of the issues surrounding the fear of childbirth are because we don't have access to experienced birthing women anymore. We don't live on farms nowadays and see animals give birth or hear family members having babies. Consequently there's a lack of knowledge, understanding and education.

Years ago a baby would be born at home and the women from the village would come. It wasn't hidden away. Childbirth is now shrouded in secrecy and the only images we have of labour are depicted on the television, where a woman is lying flat on her back screaming her head off. That is going to play a part in society's perceptions while increasing the levels of misunderstanding of how childbirth can be.

People are losing understanding of their bodies as time goes on. Most people get out of bed, sit down to have breakfast, then sit down in a car on their way to work and after all that sitting - spend more time sitting on a chair in the office! There isn't the same kind of muscle control, flexibility or strength anymore due to our sedentary lives so it's no wonder that birth has become unnatural too.

An osteopath will make adjustments to the woman's back, pelvis and hips which create space for the growing baby, ensuring she is more comfortable and the baby is in a good birth pose early on.

In the early days manipulations can be made to the internal organs which will help ailments such as indigestion. Towards the end they can work on the pelvic bowl; if the pelvis is lined up correctly delivery may be easier.

Good posture is vital to keep general aches and pains at bay for the mother-to-be - but the mother's posture also affects the position of the baby and how it lies in the womb.

Caesareans can undoubtedly save lives but they are over-used and we need to change this. We are designed to give birth and if there wasn't so much fear and worry about childbirth it would still be the natural process it used to be. The body prepares itself for labour throughout the pregnancy so a section is much more of a shock to the baby and the mother's body too than a normal birth.

The pelvis has prepared to open up for birth, but when the baby is born by caesarean the pelvis hasn't had the chance to do the job it was preparing for. This can cause post-delivery pelvic problems and also back issues.

However, giving birth isn't easy. Although a normal labour is always better, there is blood and pain and a woman needs to be prepared for the true picture of that. You shouldn't have a romantic notion of it. I think that is potentially damaging.

Babies are different according to how they've been born too. I've noticed through my own observations that a baby born normally is more of a fighter; they've had to be as they've fought their way into the world. The pain is what makes them want to live and you carry that with you through life. A baby born via section is often more jumpy and startles more easily. This may have an effect on their later life and development; physically, emotionally and socially."

© 2012 Richard Whitworth

Every birth is a very different experience and even if you've had more than one child each labour may still have some surprises in store. So, how do women succinctly define giving birth?

"Simply incredible and I wouldn't change a thing." **Catherine**

"The best day of my life as I met the (little) man of my dreams!" **Donna**

"The most amazingly empowering and special experiences of my life." **Tamandra**

"It hurts." **Amanda**

"It made me feel like the cleverest woman on the planet... to produce such magic and beauty. I felt like nobody else had ever experienced what I had! Also I was surprised at the unconditional love that happened upon me from out of the blue!" **Denise**

"Momentous – and addictive!" **Zoe**

"Surprisingly not too bad and very swift." **Rachel**

"Absolutely magical. Flipping hard work, but WOW!" **Gemma**

"A doddle compared to bringing the buggers up!" **Chantal**

"Worth it! Amazing, frightening, totally different each time, empowering and in a strange way reassuring – that my body knew what to do." **Victoria**

"Hotly anticipated, painful, frightening, yet very exciting. A special day, over quickly, readily forgotten and the result is amazing." **Kelly**

"Bloody hard work, extremely primal and the journey that turns you from a woman into a mummy" **Lisa**

"Wonderfully unique and I've had four children. It's just awesome and the most rewarding thing I've ever done. It's worth every minute of the hard work". **Shelley**

"Soon forgotten." **Vivienne**

"The end of my pregnancy and the beginning of falling in love with my perfect, beautiful baby. And it still felt the same with number four!" **Paula**

I Wish I'd known that... Tips Please!

When chatting to female friends and family it's a good idea to get their top tips. Sometimes a person may say something that totally resonates with you, and that one thing could make all the difference to you when the time comes.

Personally, my top tip for labour is to move around as much as possible - and trust your body as it knows what to. Equally for motherhood – relax and know that you're doing a good job. Yes it's easier said than done, but if that is your general ethos it will get you through.

Some top tips include

"Bring your own pillows into hospital – the ones they have are as flat as pancakes!" **Maria**

"When going into labour make sure you have someone with you who will support you completely, rub your back, and say kind and encouraging words to you. You will most likely find this one of the (if not the) most challenging things physically that you will do in your life. People don't climb Everest solo, and there's a good reason for that!" **Karen**

"Don't listen to people who harp on about how bad, terrifying, painful or long labour and childbirth is. Mums have a vague idea it's going to hurt so why do some people insist on giving them details of their horrendous ordeals? Take it as you find it... a bit painful, but mostly enjoyable and very magical." **Abigail**

*"I had a photo of my daughter to focus on and with each contraction I looked right into her eyes and breathed deeply until the pain went away. It really

helped me to stay calm and in control. I kept telling myself that this pain doesn't go on forever and you get a beautiful baby at the end." **Kelly**

"My advice to someone about to go into labour would be listen to your own body and take the pain relief you need. No one will criticise you for how you gave birth all they will do is rejoice in your new family and welcome your baby! There is no competitiveness in labour!" **Taryn**

"Being induced doesn't work if your body isn't ready. You don't HAVE to do what the doctors tell you." **Amber**

"Don't listen when they say to pack an overnight bag. I did that and ended up staying in for ten days – so always pack a bit more as if you send your husband home to get your bits you know he'll end up bringing the wrong stuff back. Also labour and birth can happen very quickly, so don't pin all your hopes on that all important birthing plan as you may not even have time to find it let alone put it into practice!" **Dawn**

"When you push it is exactly the same action as pushing out a very constipated, enormous and painful poo." **Tamandra**

*1. If you have gas and air, sip water in-between each contraction as it really dries your mouth.
2. Wax/shave your bikini line when you are due. Not only for vanity reasons, but afterwards if you have any stitches or bleeding it is nicer to be erm... trim down there!
3. Stay relaxed through your labour. The moment you start to panic or get scared it makes the pain and experience much worse.*

4. I would say the most important thing to remember is to BREATHE during your labour. Calm, gentle breathing was great for me.
5. Make sure you go out for meals, go to the cinema, have a Sunday lunch at the pub before the baby is born as you just don't have the freedom to do it afterwards.
6. Make meals and freeze them for after the birth. When you're looking after a newborn and recovering, believe me, cooking is the last thing you want to do! So to be able to zap a home cooked frozen meal in minutes is heaven!
7. Keep a pregnancy diary. I love looking back on mine and reading how I was feeling and I took pictures of my growing bump every week.
8. Don't go mad buying clothes for newborn and 0-3 months. I found that all I wanted my son to be in was sleep suits as he looked so much more comfy in them than clothes (and they sleep a lot!)
9. Do your pelvic floor exercises. I swear that doing them was the reason I recovered so quickly. I used to do them while I watched EastEnders so that I made sure I was doing them regularly.
10. Do not plan how you would like the birth to be, it will not happen that way! My advice is to keep an open mind on what will happen and just say to yourself that you will embrace whatever happens.
Stacy

Part Four

The Stories

There are many factors that make having a baby a positive experience – or not in some cases - and most women usually have a story to tell when they've been through labour.

I've been lucky enough to have collected some wonderful stories from friends, family members, clients and beyond... and am honoured to be able to share them with you.

Every single one has touched me in some way. I've cried, shivered inside and been genuinely humbled when I read the love spilling out from the words. It's been a real honour ladies thank you.

I hope that you, the reader, can take something away from the words of other women who are just like you and me.

However, one point I'd like to make is that no matter how many books you read, or how many different people you speak to your birth will be unique – and your birth story will be yours alone.

Kelly on the birth of Drew

> *"My partner was in the middle of setting up a new business and I had just managed to get another job after being made redundant.*
>
> *Although the baby was planned, we didn't think we'd be successful so quickly.*
>
> *I was a lot more tired and busy second time round, I didn't spend ages stroking my bump and talking to my*

unborn baby as I had the first time. On the positive side, I had a much better experience with my son.

I was just 36 weeks when my waters broke late on Wednesday evening. I went into hospital and assumed I would be sent home with a date for induction if nothing happened in 24 hours.
However, I was admitted as I was contracting quite regularly. I was examined and was only 2cm dilated with a bag of fluid hanging at the bottom of the cervix which meant that the baby's head could not exert enough pressure on the cervix to bring labour along. They decided to break the bag (easier said than done, it was a really unpleasant experience) and wait to see what happened.

The contractions kept coming but I wasn't progressing so they put me on a hormone drip to intensify them. That brought things along really quickly and an hour later my little boy was born.

The first stage of labour was a mere 40 minutes and the second stage only 19 minutes. I started with a TENS machine and then had gas and air. Physically I felt fine throughout but was gutted that I had to be monitored throughout due to the hormone drip so I couldn't stay active.

My labour was very controlled second time round and a really positive experience, when I finally saw my little boy I fell in love immediately - that was the emotional high of the pregnancy and an emotion I didn't feel after my first delivery – which had been very long and hard.

I feel so different about giving birth now."

Tamandra shares her experiences of giving birth to both her children Florence and Frederick

"I was on my honeymoon when I became pregnant and although the baby was planned as I'd stopped taking the pill, I didn't expect to get pregnant in the first month!

I read a couple of books which dealt with different birth stories and I read a couple of books on the early months of coping with a new baby and how to breastfeed. I had regular reflexology treatments throughout and did lots of walking.

While I loved being pregnant there was one particular time when I remember being totally overwhelmed at how much my life was going to change and it seemed as though I was alone in that (I felt that none of my family really understood that).

I had a lot of support while I was pregnant from friends and family and also my midwife. I saw the same midwife from the moment I fell pregnant until my very last appointment and she was also the first to come and see me at home with the baby.

On the day that Florence was born, I had a bath to wash my hair and found it very difficult to lean back as my bump had suddenly got very hard and solid. Ten minutes after the bath I felt a sharp pain but thought it was just a twinge.

I had my first definite contraction downstairs and remember feeling really excited. I had planned to walk lots when I started getting contractions so promptly ordered my mum to walk up the road with me.

We set off but within five minutes I was really struggling with the pain and wanted to get home so promptly ordered mum to stop talking to the neighbours and come back with me!

Things became very intense very quickly. I tried to time the contractions and they were already coming every four minutes and lasting 20 seconds (this wasn't in the books!)

I tried phoning the birthing unit and found it hard to speak but because I was still in the first hour she said I would have a while so to try and hang on as much as I could. At this point I was finding it very difficult to deal with the pain.

I phoned my husband Jim and told him to come home (he was 40 minutes away) I was insistent that I was not leaving for the unit until he got back.

The pain was overwhelming and I was frightened as I couldn't seem to calm down and work my way through it.

Throughout this time my mum and I agreed it would be good to paint my toe nails (no I don't know why either!) and actually it was funny and meant that we were giggling as my mum crawled around after me between contractions trying to finish my right foot!

By the time Jim got back I was bleeding quite heavily. I had to wait for a couple of contractions before I could even consider getting into the car.

When I arrived at the unit the midwives asked how long I had been in labour (three hours) and were quite relaxed about it all. They said that they thought I had a while to go until they checked me and told me I was fully dilated and that the baby was going to be here very soon.

However, things slowed up so much that the midwives called an ambulance to take me to the main hospital. When the ambulance people arrived and knocked on the door I told them in no uncertain terms that I was not going anywhere. I was having my baby here!

Throughout this I remained on my feet either walking around or in deep squats. Eventually I moved on to the bed and lay on my left with Jim supporting my right leg. At this point I closed my eyes and disappeared right inside myself. I distinctly remember talking to my baby at this time and taking three very slow deep breaths and telling her they were for her and I would see her very soon. At 15.10 Flo was born weighing in at 7lbs 11oz.

I felt absolute invincibility at the moment of birth and knew I'd be able to do it again and I did three years later when I had my son Freddie and I had an equally inspiring birth with him."

Onto Fred...

"Florence was three years old and I was working full time when I fell pregnant with my second child. I did a lot less preparation as we already had all the paraphernalia. I still had reflexology regularly but didn't do as much walking as I did with my first pregnancy. I had been doing yoga and so switched to pregnancy yoga. I also listened to a hypnosis-for-birth CD a number of times.

There were fewer peaks and troughs in this pregnancy but I used to worry a lot about how I would be able to maintain the equilibrium I had established with one child with now having two. I was also hyper-aware of enjoying every last minute of this pregnancy as we don't plan on having any more children. I was far more tired and ended up taking iron supplements as at one point my iron levels dropped.

In contrast to my first pregnancy I was the only person I knew who was pregnant at the time but my husband continued to support me.

There is a LOT less fanfare about your second pregnancy though and an expectation that life continues apace around you.

I think I felt that with another baby on the way this would perhaps make me feel like a "grown up" mum? There were times I was afraid of being able to cope with two children with differing demands of being able to give my daughter the same care and attention whilst also looking after the demands of a new born baby. I was especially concerned about the night time routine and also the logistics of fitting another child into our house!

I realised I was in labour when I awoke at 3am to go to the loo and couldn't stop. I sat there for ages waiting and using up no end of loo roll. My husband Jim came in when he realised I was not in bed and when I told him I thought my waters had broken he gave me the biggest hug and told me how excited he was. I popped in a pad and went back to bed. It was an anti-climax when I woke up in the morning and realised that I wasn't having any contractions and nor did I feel close to having any. I was gutted.

We went to the birthing unit and I was monitored. I got very upset when my waters broke again at the unit all over the floor.

The baby was fine but I was told that if I didn't go into labour naturally within 24 hours I had to go to the main hospital at 7am the next morning and be induced (exactly what I didn't want to happen). I was very, very depressed all afternoon as I felt I had failed (yes I know) in my pregnancy.

I had an emergency acupuncture appointment and long warm baths all in an attempt to get the contractions going but in the end I sat in the bath and sobbed my heart out in the knowledge that I was going to have to go to the hospital in the morning.

I was very nervous driving to the hospital but got so many text messages of love and support from all my friends which made such a difference (thank you).

When I got to the hospital I was in a room with three other mums and the midwife came and introduced herself and explained what would happen. She wanted to give me a cannula but I didn't want to have one in my hand as a friend had said that it hurt her hand during her active labour. I was talked into it but felt quite pressurised.

My husband found it hard to understand why I wasn't just accepting everything they said, but we talked about it and he was very supportive. I had had a great pregnancy thus far, they had told me and the baby was fine. I had a pessary inserted and was told to go and have a walk as it would take a while to get going and I may even need a further pessary. We walked around the hospital and Jim got a coffee and a newspaper. I made a call to my mum to let her know what was happening. I felt a bit tired and thought that there could be a very long day ahead so I should rest.

We went back up to the room and I read for a little bit. Jim decided he wanted to go and get something to eat and I said fine we'll have ages yet. Of course five minutes after he went I had my first contraction so I breathed through it and felt thought smugly, "Ha! I can do this lying down!" That lasted for two contractions before I had to sit up and take notice. I maintained my breathing but knew I needed to move. I started pacing up and down the corridor. I had sent Jim texts by this stage saying he needed to come back. I was walking and walking and felt quite alone and none of the staff who passed me even acknowledged me with a look let alone to ask if I was okay.

In the end the pain was becoming too much and I grabbed the next person who passed me and said that I thought I needed some help. Suddenly everything swung into motion. All my things were moved into a private room I was shown how to use the gas and air (I hadn't got on with it on my first labour). This time I found it helped me to concentrate on my breathing as the noise the breath made as you use the apparatus changes. The midwife complimented me on my breathing and that enabled me to keep going.

The pain was far sharper than with my first pregnancy and seemed a lot angrier. Jim suddenly appeared looking very worried as he had returned to the original room to find all my stuff gone. He had only been gone 10 minutes and in that time I had gone from lying peacefully reading my book to being on the bed shouting that I was ready to push. Poor chap! Again he instinctively knew what I wanted and when the midwife repositioned his hand to massage my lower back I growled at her and told her to leave him alone he knew what he was doing (which he did).

Less than 45 minutes after my first contraction I gave birth on my knees holding onto the back of the bed. It took a couple of seconds before my baby boy made any noise and I didn't dare turn around to look at him until I heard him shout. The room seemed to disappear in those seconds whilst I waited to hear his shout.

I felt triumphant and energised at that point. If I could change anything it would be that I desperately didn't want to have my baby in a hospital and whilst "all's well that ends well" I would have stood my ground and waited until I went into labour naturally as 90% of women go into labour naturally within 48 hours of their waters breaking."

Liz on the birth of Billy

"I was just about to turn 30, recently married, working full-time in a relatively successful job. I had a full and active life with a good circle of friends. I guess overall I was in a good place (although there were some relationship issues that I chose to ignore). My husband Martin and I had discussed children early on in our relationship and have both agreed we would try as soon as we got married. We married in December and I was pregnant the following April.

While I was pregnant I read up extensively on babies and childbirth and also sought advice from my close friends, which with hindsight I'm not sure is a good idea. I followed all conventional medical advice, had all the tests and scans, did antenatal classes and attended pregnancy yoga. I did very little preparation for life after birth other than to make the practical arrangements such as organising the nursery and buying clothes. I tried to discuss finances and working arrangements but felt unsupported in this regard and in the end just thought I would 'see how I felt' after the baby came.

I was totally delighted to be pregnant and embraced the whole experience. I enjoyed my bump and thinking about what the future held. I loved discussing things with my family and friends - being pregnant made me feel healthy and in some way very special.

However, I used to worry there would be something wrong with the baby, or that something would happen to me in labour. I was apprehensive about how we would manage financially because I felt a responsibility to continue contributing in this regard and was terrified that I wouldn't want to leave my baby when the time came. I had support from my husband Martin and a little from my mum, but it wasn't how I imagined it to be. I guess too much rested on Martin and with hindsight the poor man probably didn't know what to do with me!

I was determined to stay true to myself, I was concerned that I would just end up overweight and middle-aged if I didn't stay focused on trying to be the sort of mum I wanted to be. Looking back, I fought too hard to not follow the 'norm' and not be the 'typical' mum. I tried to lose weight too quickly, tried to avoid the mother and baby groups and then wondered why I was overly tired and lonely!

I went into labour on Sunday but the contractions were very mild and slow so we went to Greenwich for a long walk and ate huge pieces of chocolate cake!

I then laboured at home for several hours until I could bear it no more and we went to hospital. I was 4cm when they examined me and felt very positive and calm at this stage.

I was determined to have as natural a birth as possible, and instantly sorted out a 'route' in my room for me to pace round (a technique my then yoga teacher had suggested). It worked well and I paced round and round for several hours - I used the yoga ball and the mat, and things went well. At 6cm I started having gas and air which I had said I was happy to use in my birth plan. It was suggested to me that I should take a bath, which I tried, but the position was dreadfully painful so I got straight out! I was sick several times around this stage as the pain was so intense. Gas and air helped but the pain was still incredible.

I got through to being fully dilated but then the fun began!!! I pushed for two hours on all fours, and whilst his head was at my cervix I just couldn't get him out. I was exhausted and in so much pain by this stage.

The consultant came several times, and in the end decided that I was going to have to go in for a section. I was devastated and asked if there was anything more we could try. He agreed we would have one more attempt but that the baby's heart rate was falling so we would have to go to theatre if it didn't work.

So legs in stirrups and a ventouse on his head we went for it and amazingly he came out. The nurse had turned the ventouse up too much and there was a concern that his head was fractured – luckily it wasn't – but there was a lot of fuss and stress for a few minutes - not to mention a lot of stitches for mummy!

Once I knew he was okay, I felt incredibly elated, overjoyed, relieved, amazed and grateful. I was in awe at the beauty of my little boy and what my body had just done!"

Rebecca on the birth of Isobel

"I was working as a freelance writer and recently married when my husband Andrew and I found out we were pregnant – on New Year's Eve.

I did some antenatal yoga, listened to a hypnobirthing CD and attended NCT classes. I had a lot of support from my husband and mother and was convinced that being a mum would be hard work – and it is.

I had times when I would worry about not being able to cope or of developing postnatal depression or feeling on my own.

My waters broke at 5.30am, three days after my due date. We had been out for a spicy meal the night before at a Caribbean restaurant and I'd had my very first cup of raspberry leaf tea the day before. I couldn't believe it was happening.

Where I live, you have to go into the hospital when your waters break to make sure it's definitely happened. We were really excited - driving through the deserted London streets playing music - Biffy Clyro's Bubbles on repeat.

Once we arrived it was a bit of anti-climax. The midwife checked that my waters had broken but didn't even examine me - she just said it was a first baby so I would be ages.

She said that if I hadn't gone into labour within 24 hours they would induce me. We left and went to McDonald's for a McMuffin on the way home.

We got home and Andrew went back to bed. I took a couple of paracetamol and had a warm shower.

I rang my mum who lives in Cornwall and she started the journey up as I wanted her there at the birth. I also spoke to my sister on the phone. She has had three kids and guided me through a couple of contractions.

It wasn't long before Andrew came downstairs and it became clear that things were moving along quite fast

- the contractions were coming every few minutes. I went into the kitchen and stood by the sink. I had the TENS machine on which help distract from the pain and Andrew rubbed my back while I moved around. I couldn't believe how intense the pain was - but how it totally disappeared between contractions.

Then I felt the need to push. I went into the downstairs toilet on my own and started pushing. I felt waves of sweat wash over me - it sounds odd but they were very cooling and soothing. It felt natural, like a part of the process.

Andrew rang the hospital. This was at about 11'ish. We couldn't believe it had happened so fast.

They told him to bring me in immediately. We had a slightly surreal drive through Camden on Saturday lunchtime. I was screaming in the back seat, holding on to the arm handle and pushing.

We parked outside the hospital but getting up to the ward wasn't the easiest as the contractions were coming thick and fast.

Once up there, I went into another toilet while Andrew found a midwife. I shut myself in (I felt the need to be private) and was yelling at the top of my lungs. Someone told Andrew, 'Your wife is having a baby in the toilet.' He eventually found a midwife and took me into a room where I was finally examined.

The midwife told me that my baby was coming now. She said I could have gas and air but that it might slow things down so I decided not to. She talked me through the contractions.

The last bit was really painful as there didn't seem to be any break between the contractions.

And then she was out. We didn't know the sex but Andrew was the first to see and said, 'It's a girl.' We put her on my chest and she started feeding straight away.

Unfortunately my mum didn't arrive in time for the birth - she was on the motorway when it happened - but she came to the hospital as soon as she could.

Because it had been so quick, I couldn't believe it had happened. I was elated and shocked in equal measure.

I don't think I realised before the birth how different all babies are. I thought they were all much the same but each baby is so much an individual from day one. If there's one thing I wish I'd known, it was that."

Samantha on the birth of Grace

"Nick and I had been together for six years when he proposed on Xmas day 2007. By the time the New Year came round we started trying for a baby.

We decided that we didn't want to put any pressure on ourselves so didn't tell anyone that we were trying as we were happy that it would just happen when our time was right... so we were shocked and over the moon when we found out I was pregnant 10 weeks later! I thought it really was meant to be, and of course Nick was very proud of himself!

I looked after myself by taking all the recommended supplements and avoiding all the food I should which was really hard as I love pate and prawns! I already went to yoga so I stared going to pregnancy yoga which was great. I loved talking to all the other mums to be and exchanging stories. I really do believe that going to yoga during my pregnancy helped with the birth.

It was so exciting to tell everyone, in particular our parents. My Mum burst into tears! I loved being pregnant and have so many lovely memories of such a special time. Everyone was so happy for us, both our parents helped out massively with buying all the bits we needed and couldn't stop buying clothes. Our friends were also very excited for us as I was the first in our group to become pregnant, about two months after my best friend Emma found out she was expecting too which was great as we could talk non-stop about babies together without boring the pants off everyone else which I was always so conscious of doing!

Grace Ava Stevens was born three days early at 11:45am on Monday 10th November 2008 and weighed 6lb 02oz and I can honestly say hand on heart that it was the happiest and proudest day of my entire life to date. Any preconceptions I had about this perfect little baby I was sure we were going to have didn't even come close when the day actually arrived.

I woke up around 2.00am with a bit of a tummy ache, after a while, I gave Nick and nudge, he isn't good at being woken up so said, 'don't worry, go back to sleep.' For the next hour the pains intensified.

By the time Nick woke up I was standing up leaning over the window ledge. He jumped out of bed and grabbed a pad and pen and started recording how far apart the contractions were.

We were really worried about going to the hospital too early and getting turned away so we held out as long as we could at home, I had a bath which seemed to make the contractions stop until I got out and they were stronger than ever. Nick phoned the hospital and they asked to speak to me, I must have sounded in a lot of pain as they told us to come straight in.

The short car journey to the hospital was at 8:30am on a Monday morning in rush hour, was awful and very embarrassing – especially when you stop at lights while screaming through a contraction only to see the man in the car beside you staring at you with his mouth open!

When we got to the hospital and I was examined, I was asked if I wanted to push. I assumed she was mad as I thought I had hours to go yet, but she said I was already 8cm's and was rushed straight to a delivery room.

I managed on gas and air which worked a treat, I spent most of the time kneeling and leaning over the back of the bed, a position that I was told about at pregnancy yoga which really helped. I don't know why but I had thought that the contractions would be the hardest bit and that pushing part wouldn't be too bad, it turns out that I got that completely wrong... it was the most painful part and it seemed to take ages!

My Mum arrived not long before the pushing started and I actually remember screaming something like 'no it really won't fit!!' I remember everyone getting very high pitched and excited when they could see the baby's head and saying that it had lots of hair, and everyone was shouting push!

When she finally came out Nick said 'Sammy it's a girl!' I can't remember ever being so happy, and so proud. I couldn't wait for everyone to see our beautiful little girl."

Marianne on the birth of Megan

"I was splitting my time between living with my partner Anthony and my parent's house. We were both working full time. Anthony had bought an old Victorian house that needed a full renovation.

When I found out I was pregnant I knew I wanted to know the facts about pain relief and the side effects – but I didn't want to go to antenatal groups as didn't want to hear anything negative. The house project kept me fit. I also went on the cross trainer every night and I was very careful about eating for two as didn't think it was necessary.

I really enjoyed being pregnant and felt great. I was more scared first time round as didn't know what to expect from birth – or motherhood. I also had the occasional worry about the baby being okay.

Both my babies were breech until 36 weeks and I was dreading being forced into a caesarean. I was quite strong minded through my first pregnancy in particular and I didn't want support or advice from anyone. That changed second time round and I allowed my parents to help when I needed them.

I remember feeling very overwhelmed at times about the massive responsibility of being a parent – and knowing that once I had that baby he or she would be with me forever. Knowing I would be responsible for them for the rest of their lives scared me sometimes.

I went into labour in the evening and was very unsure of how long to wait before going to the hospital.

We eventually left for the hospital and I was 2cms upon arrival. I was very uncomfortable and the labour ward was packed with screaming mums-to- be which was really disconcerting. I was monitored from the start and wish I'd been more insistent about being mobile. One midwife said the baby was spine to spine which I know makes it more painful. Because things weren't progressing as quickly as they would have liked the doctor told me I'd need help getting the baby out and that there was no way I'd be able to push the baby out.

That motivated me, and I thought I'll show you and I did. I pushed Megan out and after she was born, I immediately asked for a phone! I felt amazing, ecstatic – I really could do anything!

When I emailed my sister a photo of me and newly born Megan she replied "You look like you could power the National Grid."

Liz on the birth of George

"Like most first time mums, the initial experience of giving birth was pretty terrifying. I am not somebody who finds it easy to relax at the best of times - but if you throw in painful contractions and an impending realisation that you actually have to get this baby out somehow – anxiety levels can (and did!) rocket! Unfortunately this did not make for a very 'relaxed' birthing experience with my first son. Drugs and some intervention were required to bring him into the world.

I was determined to aim for a much more 'relaxed' labour and birthing experience when I was pregnant

> with my second son. And so it was that I turned to pregnancy yoga. The movements and positions were similar to regular yoga, but with less intensity (depending upon how pregnant you are) and with more focus upon deep breathing and finding comfortable positions to help baby and you during labour.
>
> Although I am a born cynic (and sceptic!), I truly believe that it is only through having attended the pregnancy yoga classes that I was able to deliver my second son so quickly and efficiently.
>
> The breathing techniques learnt during pregnancy yoga, along with the positions that help to 'open the cervix', meant that I basically laboured at home.
>
> Upon reaching hospital I was found to be 9cms dilated and so was whisked straight through to the delivery room whereupon George arrived about 40mins later!
>
> Pregnancy yoga definitely taught me how to relax using controlled breathing, making me feel as though I was in control of the pain. In addition to this, I was actually able to give birth in one of the positions that we had used regularly in the classes. And so it was that my second experience of labour and birth was much easier and altogether less terrifying."

Lisa on the birth of her first baby Edward

> "I was fairly career motivated working as a qualified Chartered Accountant and Tax Adviser for an accounting practice.

However, upon starting to try for a family in late 2007 going into 2008 my career became less important as time passed.

My husband and I couldn't conceive naturally so had four attempts at IVF before I had a successful pregnancy.

It was a life changing experience and it makes you realise how special a gift a healthy baby is. When I became pregnant I went to pre-natal yoga, Pilates, NCT classes, reflexology and hypnobirthing. I also read everything I could. I loved being pregnant even though I put on too much weight and had terribly swollen ankles. I loved having a bump and feeling the baby move.

I had some pre-conceptions about having a baby, probably because we'd wanted one for so long. I thought it would be a bed of roses being a mum and so wonderful all the time. Don't get me wrong it is amazing and I love every minute, but there are some very challenging and difficult times. The thought of looking after a baby who trusts in you and relies upon you 24/7 was a bit scary at times.

I had a very quick labour. I had been out for lunch with a friend and then out walking in the afternoon with my mum when I felt my tummy tightening, so I drove home at about 5pm. I called my husband Richard to return from work and he arrived two hours later, by which point I thought I was in labour.

I called the hospital where I was told I was in the early stages of labour and to take some Paracetamol and have a bath. I took the advice having a bath, but I had one contraction in the bath and had to get out as it was so painful. I used my TENS machine and focused on my breathing as the contractions were becoming more frequent and stronger.

About 9.45pm I called the hospital again and they said I seemed to be dealing very well and I could remain at home. However, I knew I needed to go to hospital so we made our way there. Before we left, I had a show and felt the sensation to push so for the whole car journey to hospital I had to use my breathing to stop myself.

We arrived at the hospital at 11pm where I was examined and was told I was 8cm dilated and it would be a few more hours. Shortly afterwards my waters broke and I remember the midwife asking how I wanted to give birth as this baby was coming!

I gave birth on all fours and within a few pushes my beautiful baby boy was born at 11.45pm.

I felt amazing - it was a wonderful experience. I was so proud to be a mummy.

My husband was very good and supportive throughout my pregnancy and during the IVF. He was my birth partner and did fantastically standing beside me as I gave birth."

The thing that shaped my birth experience...

> *"For me pregnancy yoga rocked – and made both my birth experiences positive."* **Liz**

> *"Understanding exactly what was happening at every single stage."* **Catherine**

> *"The wonderful team that carried out my section meant I was calm and relaxed throughout – as was my husband."* **Louise**

> *"My wife had a really hard labour first time round and was so scared when she was pregnant again. However, I was so proud of her as she did a lot to help herself. She attended antenatal yoga and practiced her breathing every single day at home. To be honest I used to tease her as I wasn't sure how much it would help. I can say that second-time-round it was effortless and she didn't have any pain relief at all. She just breathed through the contractions and it was over in under three hours. I couldn't believe it."* **Dave**

However your baby came into the world will fade into insignificance in time as you go on the next phase of your journey – mothering your child. In time the discomfort and pain will seem a distant memory and instead you'll be facing a whole new load of new and wonderful experiences.

But, it's important to acknowledge any feelings or issues that you have about your baby's birth. If you're experiencing any flashbacks or negative emotions speak to somebody about it. Nobody is going to judge you and if you deal with things as they come up – as soon as they come up - it will be easier in the long run. Sometimes just acknowledging feelings to a family member or friend is enough, but if not have a chat to your health visitor or doctor and see what they suggest.

Let's hear it from the boys

So what is it like to see the woman you love go through pain, give birth and ultimately become a mother? Here some brave men share their experiences about birth and fatherhood

Angus shares his experiences of the night that baby Kieran was born. It was quite traumatic, but luckily there was a happy ending. It just goes to show that you can't plan everything...

> "I woke up in the middle of the night and realised my wife Sophie was in labour. She told me she needed to get to the hospital.
>
> We've got four other children and they'd all come early and Sophie always has quick labours so it was imperative to get a move on.
>
> By the time we got downstairs to the kitchen, Sophie was very agitated and kept shouting something wasn't right and asked me to call an ambulance.
>
> After that she fainted and started to lose some blood. It was terrifying and I didn't know what to do. Even though we've got four other children, they've all been born in hospital where you're properly monitored.
>
> To see my wife in a heap on the kitchen floor was very scary. I phoned for an ambulance and was told one was on its way – but the operator told me not to get off the phone; that's when it dawned on me - I was going to deliver the baby.
>
> Sophie came round again and started screaming before she fell silent – she'd blacked out again.

I went over and could see the baby's head coming out, I threw the phone on the floor as the head was blue and I could see the cord was wrapped around its neck. As more of the baby emerged the cord became tighter. I pushed the baby up and untangled the cord, which felt like a giant rubber band. I wasn't thinking, adrenaline took over and I was acting on instinct. Once I'd untied the cord I picked the phone up to tell the operator what had happened.

While I was talking Sophie delivered the rest of the baby.

I was holding the baby in one hand and the phone in the other. The baby was born within 10 minutes. When the baby was born I assumed he was dead because he wasn't moving or crying.

Sophie had gone into herself, and wasn't saying anything. I rubbed the baby's back and gently shook him to see if that would help. I prayed he wasn't dead. It felt like hours but it was probably only a few seconds before he started to move and breathe. It was a miracle and I can honestly say I'm a different man. You think you know what's important until life teaches you otherwise.

Our eldest daughter Lorna, who's 12, came into the kitchen as the head was emerging and sat on the floor and held her mum's hand. She was so calm – unlike me, who was crying and a bit hysterical.

By the time baby Kieran was born all the children were downstairs. George who's five had a cuddly toy for his new brother. We gave the children jobs to do.

George and Ruby, who's nine went to get towels and Leon who's 10 fetched some cushions so we could wrap the baby up and get Sophie a bit more comfortable.

We were all shell-shocked. 25 minutes after Kieran was born, who weighing a tiny 5.05lb's the ambulance crew arrived. They told us it was a job for the midwife so rang for one, with the baby still attached to Sophie by the umbilical cord.

We waited on the kitchen floor for the midwife who took a further 45 minutes to arrive. When she did, she delivered the placenta and cut the cord with a pair of scissors.

Once that was done we made our way to the hospital to get checked over, as Kieran was pre-term. Luckily Sophie and the baby have been given a clean bill of health.

We know how lucky we've been. We could have had a very different outcome but the end result is a very calm, relaxed baby who's absolutely lovely. We'll tell him about his very dramatic birth when he's old enough."

Publisher and Father of three David shares his thoughts on Fatherhood

"I became a father at what I consider to be at an early age. I was 27 and had been married for 18 months. We had planned to have children, just not quite then, and so it all came as something of a shock.

In the months leading up to his birth, I felt little. The bump kicked, my wife was obviously changing physically and mentally and something was definitely going to happen, but I just could not envisage what. I seemed to be emotionally detached from the impending event and felt barely old enough to be responsible for my own life, yet alone someone else's, a baby, a son. In retrospect, that detachment was utterly down to my own immaturity.

My wife was taken in to hospital a week or so before she was due because there were possible complications. It was a tough time for both of us, especially as you'd end up chatting to other pregnant women on the ward who were very happy to share some pretty revolting gynaecological details with you. Dawn was then allowed home and I remember we celebrated with a mighty steak dinner.

Her waters broke in the flat and we phoned the hospital who told us to wait. We waited until it was the middle of the night and we could wait no more. Dawn was in pain. I was utterly in control, strangely for me. I was calm and collected. The headlights of the car picked out a beautiful urban fox and I commented on it. I was a tad miffed that Dawn did not seem to share my awe of this beast. The Police stopped us as it turned out I'd left a rear door partially open. When they realised the situation they gave us a short escort.

It wasn't an easy birth and I remember thinking that I just wanted Dawn safe – forget the child. It was all too primal and painful. No I didn't want to see the baby's head. I just wanted my wife safe.

Child birth seems to me to be the perfect argument against intelligent design. It's a crazy method of bringing new life to the earth, forcing this rather large thing through an aperture that size...

When he was born I'd hoped for a sudden surge of love and joy at the event. It didn't happen. Instead I was more concerned about the blood and gore and the exhaustion my wife experienced after 18 hours in labour. This skinny, rather ugly thing with his distorted head (he'd been a forceps birth) was simply a bi-product.

Love came slowly. I bonded properly when we took him on holiday when he was three months old. He was radiant with golden hair and chubby legs. He smiled and laughed and at last when I held him in my arms I felt deep, unconditional love for him.

He's now a successful young man of 25, making his way in the world. He has a younger brother of 21 and a sister of 17. As a young dad I've been closer to them as they've grown up. Have I been a good father? Well, that question does trouble me. I think so. I've been around for them, they seem to enjoy my company and they seem to appreciate me most of the time.

I take the cynics view. There's no such thing as a perfect parent producing perfectly well-balanced children. All you can do as a father is to limit how screwed up they are. I'm happy to report my children are well adjusted, clever and fun to be around and I could not imagine my life without them. Maybe I've matured at last."

Part Six

The Early Days

So your baby has arrived – now the fun really begins. The early days are hard going as you adjust to having a new little person around. In addition you may not be feeling great either. It's crucial at this time that you don't start putting too much pressure on yourself. Try if possible to only focus on you and your baby.

Top Tips for the first few days:

- Sleep when your baby sleeps – okay you probably won't – but I'm going to say it anyway! It will make such a difference to your life. I'm a real fan of power napping and there's all kind of scientific studies that state the benefits. If you struggle to fall asleep just rest, read a book, lie down or do some yoga nidra, which is also known as dynamic sleep.
    - Lie down and allow your body to find its own natural rhythm, don't force your breath to be slow, just accept it at its own pace.
    - Once your breath has slowed focus your awareness on your body, be aware of your body sinking a little deeper into the floor upon exhalation.
    - Focus your awareness on your feet, allow your feet to become heavy and relaxed. Your feet are relaxed.
    - Now this feeling travels up your body and into your legs. Focus your awareness on your legs, allow your legs to become heavy and relaxed. Your legs are relaxed.

- Focus your awareness on your hips, allow your hips to become heavy and relaxed. Your hips are relaxed.
- Be aware of your back. Allow your big back muscles to become heavier and heavier as you breathe. Your back is relaxed.
- Focus your awareness on your shoulders – ensure there is space between your shoulders and your ears, allow your shoulders to become heavy and relaxed. Your shoulders are relaxed.
- Focus your awareness on your neck, allow your neck to become heavy and relaxed. Your neck is relaxed.
- Your chest and your tummy are lifting as you inhale. Feel your rib case lift as you breathe in. Allow your breath to deepen. Allow your chest and tummy to become heavy and relaxed. Your chest and tummy are relaxed.
- Your arms are increasingly heavy as you breathe. Your arms feel so heavy that you couldn't move them even if you wanted to. Allow any lingering tension to be released from your arms. Your arms are relaxed.
- Allow your hands to sink a little deeper into the floor beneath you. Relax your hands. Your hands are relaxed.
- Focus your awareness on your head and release any tension from your hairline. Relax your head. Your head is relaxed.
- Relax your face. Be aware of your face, ensure you're not frowning, screwing up your eyes, grinding your teeth or clenching your jaw. Your face is relaxed.

- - The whole of your body is relaxed. Your mind is relaxed. All is well.
- If you're lucky enough to have your mum around, or another close family member and they offer help – then take it.
- If you've got the money to have a cleaner and/or ironing person then book them in for at least the first month or so.
- Don't worry about entertaining guests when they arrive. Most people will understand the house is likely to be a bit of a mess and there won't be cake on offer – and if they don't understand don't worry about it.
- Accept help from your partner – or give him tasks to do if he's not that forthcoming with ideas.
- Enjoy being with your little one. Cuddle them, marvel at their brilliance and savour every single second whilst you do so.
- Don't worry that the sleepless nights and general chaos will last forever – before you know it you'll be an old-hand at this baby-lark and you'll struggle to remember what you used to do with your time before your baby was born.
- From the moment your baby is born you'll probably have set ideas about the kind of mum you want to be and the kind of baby you want too. Just remember - the things you do in the early days such as cuddling your baby to sleep have an effect on your little one so be aware of starting precedents that you're going to find hard to continue with. I've got friends who still have to lie with their head beside their child's five years on – because that's what they've always done. Of course if you're happy to do this it isn't an issue – but if you'd rather your child is able to settle

themselves, it's worth thinking carefully before you get into a routine with your baby.
- Remember - being born is hard work so for the first few days or so (and perhaps longer if you had a lot of drugs during labour) your baby will be very sleepy. This can lull you into a false sense of security and you may go into shock when they finally 'wake up'.
- Little ones tire really easily and if you're over-stimulating and passing them around to endless visitors there will probably be a fall-out – and that will probably come to a head at 3 o'clock in the morning!
- It's important for a baby to learn to settle themselves, so set them down in their own space so they can learn how to do so. If you're constantly over the top of them fussing at every stage they're not going to learn how to get to sleep without you there.
- Put them down in their own room for short periods of time. The advice is babies should sleep in their parent's room in their own cot or Moses basket for six months. However I would suggest getting them used to their own room throughout this period and putting them down for their naps in their own room as well as changing their nappy in there and occasionally playing there so they have a positive association with their own space.
- Make sure the room they're sleeping in is dark – obvious? Yes - but it makes a real difference.
- Don't react to every noise your baby makes. Spend some time observing your newborn from a distance and be aware that they make lots of noises, sighs and little whimpers without waking up – and they don't necessarily need you at that moment. If you go rushing in all guns blazing every time you hear a

snuffle, the chances are your baby will expect that from that day on.
- If you're relaxed, your baby will be relaxed too. If you're constantly fussing and worrying about your baby they will pick up on this, so try to chill out a bit. Leave them be for a while and allow them to discover their world. If you struggle with that then perhaps you could try some yoga or meditation to help.

Mark Woods has written Babies & Toddlers for Men, and shares his early experiences of fatherhood, assuring us that men do find parenting as dauntingly wonderful as women

Here's one man's guide to having a baby...

The First Day of the Rest of Your Life

The time has come to take your new family home and so begins your life as a father.

From the moment you check for the ninth time that the car seat is secured properly before you drive away from the hospital, you feel the weight of responsibility and nervousness wrestling with the giddiness of excitement and pride inside your overcrowded head.

Like the earliest people on the planet, you now live in a world of firsts; they just keep on coming and each one represents a challenge or a moment of joy (often at one and the same time) that will grab your undivided attention like you would not believe.

Bringing Baby Home

I remember thinking as I skipped into hospital swinging an empty car seat to and fro that in half an hour's time or so everything would be different.

Once you've had the obligatory GULP! moment when reality dawns that the pair of you need to immediately transform from looking after yourselves pretty badly, to taking care of someone else fantastically well, stuff begins to happen.

Feeding your baby

There's very little that's as fundamental or as emotive for you and your partner in the first few months of parenthood as the process of feeding your baby.

You'd think it would be a doddle – but it can be hard going at first while you learn what suits baby and mum too – just go with the flow and it will work out just fine.

Thriving

No matter how you decide to feed your baby you will become obsessed, consumed and just a little boring to almost everyone else on the planet about how your little one is progressing on her growth chart in her first few weeks and months.

The S Word

Sleep is going to become your new obsession.

Accept that you will be tired, accept that you will be beyond tired and accept that despite it all, you'll just have to carry on. Think of it not as something to be endured but as a rite of passage, an extreme sport to be taken on and beaten.

The First Big Cry

Crying is designed solely to grab your attention and evolution, as it has a habit of doing, has engineered it so the noise is as effective as possible at doing just that. So powerful is it in fact that some women can lactate just by hearing a cry and it doesn't even have to emanate from their baby.

So don't worry if crying gets to you, it's meant to.

The First Nasty Nappy Change

Whoever does the PR for nappy changing needs a talking to, it's not that bad.

Okay on occasion you'll put your finger in something disagreeable, but at least it's your baby's disagreeable produce. If, by some freak of nature, you are unlucky enough to find yourself changing the nappy of someone else's child you will come to see your own offspring's excrement in a whole new and favourable light.

The First Smile

Your baby's first proper social smile can occur as early as four weeks post birth – and after the month or so you and your partner will likely have had, a little bit of a reward will be gratefully received.

If, though, you are lucky enough to see a smile even earlier than the four week mark, don't let any sour faced fool dismiss it as wind – smile right back and let the love in.

Your Baby

Your little one will change from a watery eyed, floppy-limbed alien-like creature to a being capable of holding its head up, tracking objects with her eyes and even smiling at you.

Never again will they learn so much so fast. They even begin to recognise you and your partner from the six billion other people on the planet - clever.

Your Partner

For many new mothers while its undoubtedly a tough sleep-deprived time they are also experiencing the most intense and emotionally powerful period of their lives as they bond in quite spectacular fashion with their child.

This bonding process can be amazing to watch and be around, although some Dad's do report feeling a touch left out as a love affair unfolds in front of them – which leads us on to…

You

If you do feel your nose being put slightly out of joint by the closeness of the bond between mother and child know this; your time will come.

If you possibly can just revel in the moment, embrace every 3am wake up, relish every nuzzle, soak it up and file it away because the first three months are rock hard for sure, but they are also magical, unique and fleeting... Enjoy.

© 2012 Mark Woods

From mum-to-mum

From the moment you find you're pregnant you find yourself immersed in a different – and often very competitive world. It begins with the size of your bump, progresses onto how you gave birth, it then moves on to how many teeth your baby has and so it continues.

If possible try to take a step back from any competition. Just do things your way, from the way you give birth and then rear your child. Yes you'll make mistakes along the way but that's part of motherhood and the important thing is to learn from them and not to beat yourself up over being the 'perfect mother'. I'll let you into a secret. The perfect mother doesn't exist and I reckon all those 'perfect mothers' have all the same insecurities and hang ups as the rest of us.

The following women share what being a mum means for them and the things they wish they'd been told:

> *"I was lucky as I had easy, normal pregnancies and labours with both my kids. My advice to any new mum to be would be to take the whole experience one step at a time. Don't put the extra pressure on yourself to do it completely naturally- if you need the help of the drugs take them. If you have to have a section, for whatever reason then just go with it. If you can't breast feed then so be it, after all Mother Nature will always find its way, and you won't be any less of a mother to your little bundle of joy. Becoming a mum for the first time, and the second time is equally mind-blowing. The thing that hit me the most was that nobody had prepared me for falling deeply and unconditionally in love with my baby. I read all the pregnancy books but nothing stated this fact! Even*

second time around the feelings of "will I love this baby as much as my first born" becomes completely void when you see them for the first time. Sounds very cheesy but there is always more love to go round." **Bridget**

"I wish all new mums could understand just how much of what they hear from other mums is total rubbish. There is so much competition and if you're impressionable and desperate to do everything right it is damaging to listen to other mums! It should come with a health warning! Other babies sleep all night, smile from the moment they are born, breast feed with mum smiling over them serenely, walk at nine months, feed themselves at 18mths, are potty trained at two and can read bloody Biff, Chip and Kipper books before they go to school! I kid you not. New mums need to realise this is not the case and that every child is different – and every mother is different too." **Liz**

"Know that your life will change forever and that there are no prizes for doing everything yourself. It is much kinder to you and your child and indeed everyone else to share!! Share responsibility, concerns, decisions and more. When your baby is born and sleeps (which they do loads but only for a matter of weeks) YOU sleep. Don't clean the house for unnecessary visitors, iron your baby grows or try to keep up the work you were doing before. None of that matters but your health does. SLEEP or rest and do very little so your body can recover because within weeks your baby will be awake far more and you may also be breastfeeding which takes a lot of energy as

well. It is all too easy to realise too late that you have squandered your precious recovery time and that now you are simply shattered every day and there is no need for this. So, take heed! Listen to advice from everyone; other mums, your mum, your partner's mum etc. People just love to give it and often your realise you are not alone and in fact everything is perfectly normal and this gives you reassurance and strength. My lovely friend, Beryl said to me: "The good times don't last, and the bad times don't last. So enjoy the good times and don't get hung up on the bad times as with babies/children, things change constantly." This is true." **Karen**

"Share books all the time, and when the time comes for your little darling to go to school, read their reading books WITH THEM every evening. It can make all the difference in their progress. Reading underpins all learning." **Tania**

"You can love your children and still not be 'fulfilled' by only being a mother and it's okay not to enjoy the 'perfect mother role' – but find the things you all enjoy together." **Amber**

"Sleep as much as possible before your bundle of joy arrives – because you sure won't be getting any after!" **Jo**

"You will only go out for dinner or to the cinema with your husband five times in the next five years so make the most your time together as a couple before your baby arrives. Motherhood is the best thing in the world and however hard it may seem in the first few weeks it only gets better and better." **Marika**

"Once your baby is here cuddle her/him as much as possible – this does not spoil them." **Dawn**

"I wish I'd allowed myself to worry more about me. Instead I beat myself up about it and felt bad for thinking about my own feelings. I felt that I should be concentrating all my energy on my new baby. But the reality was I was scared of what I was feeling; constantly dizzy, exhausted and very sore from the stitches. I didn't know if what I was feeling was normal... but it was. And my baby was just fine, he just got on with things, fed really well, slept really well and gave me the focus to stop worrying and get on. It made me realise if he was okay after all that being born malarkey, surely I can be fine too. I'm a mum now- it's what we do right? But I think you should allow yourself to worry a bit about your own needs - after all you are the most important thing now in your baby's life and you need to be well and feeling ok." **Jo**

"I wish I had known more about looking after a newborn. I didn't put my little girl down to sleep often enough and ended up with a lot of screaming from over-tiredness! I would tell anyone just to go with the flow during labour – and that you can do it without pain relief – oh and to leave the cord once the baby is born so they get maximum blood. Have it cut once it's stopped pulsing (not a long time)." **Gemma**

"Forget about planning the birth, nature has its own plan. Keep calm and carry on. Don't compare yourself to other mothers. There are few people who tell it how it really is. The rest are just kidding themselves or pretending to be perfect. Know you're doing a good

job – because nobody else is going to tell you that you are. Really try to enjoy it because it will be over in a flash. Basically it's the best and the worst job you will ever do." **Sue**

"Being a mum can be the most challenging role you will ever do. The rewards are massive, the lows are low. But despite all that you will love them unconditionally and never be more proud than you are of your children." **Cheryl**

"It's your baby, do what you feel is right for you; whether you choose to breastfeed your baby, give them a dummy or wean them early - or not, there's no right and wrong and I don't understand why some mums look down on others for making different choices to their own." **Abi**

"Routine is the way forward – and that until three months a baby shouldn't be awake for more than about an hour and a half at a time so as not to get over tired. But the big one for me is to trust your instincts. If you think something is wrong keep pestering the doctors and don't them fob you off saying all babies cry a lot. You know your own baby. Result for me was that my youngest had a milk allergy – change of milk = happy baby." **Rachel**

"Do whatever it takes to maximize the amount of sleep you get – how much you have slept colours everything about the way you see things!

Prioritise yourself – a midwife friend of mine was insistent about this one. "There's a reason why on an aircraft you're told to fit your own oxygen mask first *before helping others," she told me. "If you can't breathe, you can't do anything for anyone else."*

Practise saying, "Yes, please" and "Thank you very much" – accepting help from others is sometimes very hard. You don't need to be in a state of desperation before you ask for or accept some support. Fortunately, this is a time when people are usually very willing to help, even if they wait to be asked rather than offer." **Alex**

Part Seven

From Me to Mummy

The fact is a woman changes when she has a baby and that's not necessarily just because her tummy will never quite be the same again. Many women who have previously been incredibly career driven suddenly realise they want an easier job that doesn't take them away from their baby too much. Other women find a sense of fulfilment they never thought possible.

No matter who you are, how much money you earn or what job you have you cannot help but be moved by giving birth– and becoming a mother.

Having a baby is so humbling – your little one doesn't care if you're an office cleaner or top lawyer. If she wants to throw up all over you or scream all night she will. We all go through the same issues no matter where we are in our lives – although of course having a house full of staff may help...

For many women relinquishing control is something they really struggle with. It may be for the first time in your adult life things don't 'go to plan'. You may have a lovely day out in mind and need to leave the house by 10.00am sharp, cue explosive nappy or projectile vomiting...

Yes it's a time that tests even the most patient of women. But the weird thing is for most women it doesn't matter. So what if you've gone from wearing Prada to Primark and have that acrid smell of stale sick hanging around you – you've had a baby!

I will never forget the night that Zak was born, he was fast asleep as was his dad but I couldn't sleep myself. I just sat and stared at him all night, counting his fingers and toes over and over again – simply marvelling at this beautiful, perfect baby that I had made and birthed all by myself. Okay so maybe I was high on the gas and air but I was just ecstatic and the feeling of love totally and utterly overwhelmed me. I knew that life would never be the same again. And do you know what? It hasn't been. It's been better.

Yes, there have times when I've cried in sheer frustration and temper – and felt like the worst mother in the world because I felt I'd got it wrong but every day my son grows I grow too and I've learnt far more from him than he'll ever learn from me.

There are so many milestones and challenges along the way and just when you've cracked one, sleeping through the night, eating solids, potty training, starting school or leaving home – another pops up to replace it. As your child grows older you really do learn not to sweat the small stuff, to choose your battles carefully and not to spend time worrying and over-analysing every single thing you and your child say, do and think.

There are always new reports in the press that worry the life out of you – take them all with a pinch of salt and try not to get drawn into panicking about every single decision you make. Sometimes, taking a step back is all you need to do to realise how ridiculous many of these claims are, by which time some other expert or other will probably have a totally different opinion anyway.

As a mother you'll never know a moment's true peace again unless your child is by your side. You will over-analyse, worry always and talk too much about your offspring. You will see the world differently and danger in places you'd never even acknowledged before. Accept it – you are different and have probably become all the things you swore you never would.

But you will find joy in places you never imagined possible and experience love in its truest and purest form. You will be happy just sitting in a chair cuddling your child or watching them sleep. A day in the park kicking leaves around gives you a bigger high than an all-night-bender (and without the hangover). When you hear stories about women running back into burning buildings to save their child it suddenly all makes sense – because you would.

We should celebrate all mothers – in whatever decisions they make. At the end of the day for the most part we're all doing the best we can in the hardest job there is. And just because another woman makes different choices to your own it doesn't necessarily means she's wrong – there's ambiguity in labour and child-rearing too and what works for one family, won't necessarily work for another. As long as a child isn't being abused or in danger nobody has the right to cast aspersions on another's choices.

Many women don't tend to feel valued in their role of mother. How many times have you asked a woman what she does for a living, only to hear her reply, "I'm just a house wife." Well hats off to those 'house wives' – because I tell you now every day I go to work is a doddle compared to spending a day at home being mum.

Gemma shares her thoughts of being a mum to her five children

> *"Having had five children you might have thought I would get used to seeing those blue lines appear, but*

no! Each time my initial thoughts were, "Oh my goodness! What have I done?" That's not to say the pregnancy was a surprise but just the enormity of what you have done starts to sink in!

Very quickly excitement takes over as you take in what will be happening. Pregnancy to me is a time of very many emotions and feelings. Sometimes all mixed together! I personally love the secrecy of it at the beginning when it is only me and my husband who know.

I never really worry about labour as I see it as something that has to be done, so worrying about it is pointless. With my first pregnancy I did start to get very nervous as the date grew nearer and did go through a stage of thinking that maybe I would just stay pregnant as it seemed easier! However, I did it and got through it. It is the most amazing, painful, emotional, scary, life- changing thing you can ever do. Unfortunately, I don't think you realise it at the time, it's afterwards when you look back it becomes real. I wouldn't say it is an enjoyable experience, just one you have to do. I was lucky that my labours were all fairly straight forward, with very little intervention or problems.

The moment you deliver your baby and see them for the first time I would say my overwhelming emotion is amazement, closely followed by love and pride. It seems impossible that you could have had this baby inside you. I wasn't scared of looking after any of my babies, I loved every second!

> That's not to say I didn't find it very hard at times and incredibly relentless, but I wouldn't have changed it for anything.
>
> It is 11 ½ years since I had my first baby and it is still relentless and very hard!! It is also wonderful. And maybe I don't say it enough, especially to my children, but I love being a mum!"

Here some women share just how having a baby has changed them

> "Motherhood is an emotional rollercoaster and a bit like the Krypton Factor! I think I cried everyday for three months after having Oliver, sometimes at stupid things (like Gok Wan's How to Look Good Naked!). I went through a phase of feeling really lonely, as I really missed my bump, I missed carrying Oliver around with me everywhere I went and it took me a while to adjust to not having him there. I remember having to reason with myself that surely it's better now he is out and I can see him and watch him change. But I did really miss that, like I had forgotten something or was missing an arm. Ultimately, after all the changing moods and challenges that you face, motherhood eventually turns into something you just do without even thinking about . It's something I look forward to experiencing more and more as each day brings something new." **Jo**
>
> "I did start to crave adult conversation and this for me was probably the hardest part of adjustment, alongside going from being financial independent with a full-time job to relying on my husband Robin financially. There were times that I felt low." **Lisa**

"Since having Olivia I have had to slow down and let go of control a lot more. I have become hugely softer. It was noted by everyone who knew me in my work – before I was a terrier, afterwards I still got results but with none of the aggression. I felt no need to prove myself to the outside world and ultimately I am more self-assured." **Nicola**

"I was ready to have a baby and ready to calm down. What I hadn't reckoned on was how much I would have to do by myself or that he wouldn't sleep. The days and nights were long and rolled into each other. These two things combined did make me feel suffocated at times, and the responsibility overwhelmed me. By the time Billy was 18 months (and still not sleeping) I began to feel a little unhinged at times. I realise now this is fairly normal but at the time thought it was only me. Being a mother has given me a sense of hope, purpose, perspective and responsibility that was never there before. It's given me happiness and a love that I have never experienced before. It's made me incredibly intolerant of bad parents and perhaps quite judgemental. I do not understand people who do not feel as I do about being a parent. I would die for my children without a moment's hesitation." **Liz**

"Seriously I always felt maternal before having my son Marley - I was so excited to be a mum. I had convinced myself he was a girl and I was gobsmacked that he wasn't. My initial thoughts were what will I do with a boy? I remember the first time I saw Marley I simply fell in love. It was instant. I couldn't believe the intensity of my feelings for him. I

was shocked by how I felt. The first night after he was born I remember looking at him and feeling scared at the thought of being responsible for him for forever. I was petrified at the thought of something going wrong. It was so intense; the worry and the instant guilt. I felt guilty about everything that I had done in my life and wanted to change and be a better person. All these thoughts were racing through my mind in an instant after he was born. I loved him so much - it was gushing love that makes you feel amazing, euphoric, scared and sick in your stomach all at the same time. Having a baby sent me on a bit of a soul searching journey and I am still discovering more about this journey. Now I have just had Rani my beautiful baby girl I feel complete. I think I have changed so much since I had Marley. The usual things have changed I have become mature, responsible and a lot more organised – although I'm still not great with routine and time keeping. One thing that has completely surprised me since I have become a parent is how much I am like my own parents. We spend all our young lives running away from what are parents are like and challenging them and rebelling against them. All the things I said when I was younger about being different with my children that I would not parent like my parents, but I have become them and I now realise why they were the way they were. It's a good thing I think. I appreciate why they were strict and hard on us. I appreciate why they would worry and most of all I appreciate why they wanted so much for me. I feel exactly the same about my children."
Amelia

"Occasionally and only fleetingly I yearn for my old life. My itchy feet for travel have gone and I no longer feel the need to travel to the ends of the earth (for now). Family is very important to me, and they are my focus, and I put Lou first. I do need time for me and I go to yoga and visit the gym regularly otherwise I'd be a crabby cow. Very small things make me feel contented, rather than always planning the next big adventure. In an ideal world I would have met Will when I was younger and had a family younger, but that can't be changed. I think I see things a bit differently now but can't quantify that. Some of my friendships have grown even stronger which is great, some have faded a bit – but that's just the way life goes." **Rachel**

"I have discovered anger that I had forgotten since childhood as my little girl taps straight into my inner child, so I can give her temper tantrums a run for their money. But she's also made me grateful for the simple pleasures in life all over again; the wonder of watching the clouds, sunshine dappling etc. I am freer with my own creativity now as Daisy shows no fear in her creations - scribbling, mixing colours and putting together things that clash and yet the end result is inspired - colourful, fresh, real. My body has changed and not for the better. Having a child late in life does mean that recovery is longer, skin is not so elastic and in the main I have had to work much harder than people ten years my junior did. I am also less selfish whilst at the same time very aware of just how selfish I am! I think of her constantly and recall waking with her on my mind when she was a few months old and realising that I was never going to just be me in my

head anymore for the rest of my life! But having a child that needs you and demands of you also highlights how much of my time and energy I am willing to give to another person and the limits can lead to guilt even though I acknowledge that they are healthy and important for both of us." **Karen**

"I now realise what is important in life. Things like work, bills, family dramas and what the neighbours are doing really does not matter. My boys are my number one priority, and it is quite scary how he consumes all my thoughts and feelings. You would do anything in the world to protect your child." **Stacy**

"Although I don't think I've changed that much as a person, my priorities are completely different now I have children in my life. I'm not as ambitious as I used to be and I want to focus on raising my kids the best way I can. Something that has surprised me is other people's reactions to us since we've had children. Some of our friends have excluded us from social events since we've had a family. That used to be quite hurtful although I've got over that now and don't want to waste time feeling bitter just because we have children and they don't." **Paula**

"I think I am more patient and being a mother has forced me to slow down to a different pace which does not come naturally. It has certainly made me a much better doctor. Without children, I don't think you can understand the level of angst you can feel, nor the guilt for well - everything really..." **Helen**

"I'm calmer and much less selfish. The world scares me more and I'm more concerned about family

relationships than I was before and less worried about money/material things.

I accept my physical defects more and acknowledge the wonderful thing my body has done by having two children which is more important than trying to look supermodel-thin all the time.

Being a mother has been the most wonderful but hardest thing I've ever done in my life. I was ambitious to be successful at work, but I now just want to be successful in this the most important job I've ever had - giving my children the very best start in life." **Kelly**

"I was ready to become a mother. However, I am so independent and love being free and impulsive. Sometimes, for a moment or two I miss my old life and travelling the world and being a free spirit but I have learnt it is possible to still be 'you' when you have a child. Being a mother is the biggest and scariest job in the world, yet it is the most rewarding at the same time. There is nothing like the bond I have with my children and I wouldn't change anything for the world!" **Caroline**

"I'm much less bothered about my career and I am happier. I simply love being a mum; I never thought I could be as fulfilled as I am." **Louisa**

"Since becoming a mother, I've changed in so many ways. Some of the most notable differences are a permanent and rather exhausting desire to protect the children from danger and/or pain, I'm much less relaxed as I always feel as if there is something which

needs doing and I have an inner strength and happiness. I also have empathy with my mother and all other mums now I know exactly how much effort is put into the most demanding and underpaid job in the world." **Louise**

"As a young mum I knew I would have different challenges ahead of me and there are times when it is really hard being a mum at 22 but seeing my little girl happy is the best feeling in the world and I am determined to give my daughter the best in life. I am far stronger than I ever realised and I wouldn't change a thing." **Hayley**

"Since I've had my daughter I'm far less selfish, and it's made me realise that the most important thing in my whole world, is my child coupled with the amazing realisation that you really can love something THAT much. Although I don't feel very different I am a bore though. I feel that there are times when I only want to talk about my precious baby, and that everyone will surely want to meet her... but then I remember she's only that special to us." **Helen**

"I feel very proud to be a mum and have grown in maturity. My outlook on life and understanding what is important has changed for the better as well." **Lisa**

"I thought the birth was the all-important moment. I had no idea that what comes after is so much more overwhelming." **Andrea**

"I have found a level of contentment that I've never experienced before and I feel the more settled than ever." **Rachel**

"I have realised how controlling I was of every aspect of my life. I needed to know what was happening in every situation. I have relaxed a lot since becoming a mum as a lot of parenting is kind of "suck it and see." You cannot control every situation. Babies may not want to sleep/feed/poo/cry/wake when you want them too, and toddlers certainly don't. But as important as I find a routine works in my life with the children, nothing is set in stone. And I don't expect anything.

I used to have extremely high expectations of myself and others and was often left disappointed if things didn't happen the way I wanted them to. A lot of people that I am friends with through motherhood would have found me very harsh and not very forgiving and probably would not have been friends with me if they had met me before having children! I would love to have 100% patience 100% of the time, but this is too high an expectation. I now spend most of time trying to be the person I would like my children to become. I have definitely become less demanding of myself and allow things to happen rather than forcing the issue on certain things. I am much more tolerant of other people's opinions than I used to be, as with parenting it is very much each person to their own as to how you deal with children and I have found that I can apply this to most other situations too, and allow people their opinions without me forcing mine on them!! With regards to pregnancy/birthing/parenting I believe that knowledge is power and the more you know the more you can mentally prepare yourself, which is a huge help when you realise you are responsible for another little life."
Tannita

"Life changes once you have a baby, I found it hard not being able to just go out at the drop of a hat – and my husband found that even harder. Nothing prepared me for the overwhelming feeling when I held my baby in my arms. I don't think I could even begin to explain. From that moment everything changed. Although I still have other goals in life, being a good mum is the most important one. My girls always come first. I am so much more confident and a great multi-tasker now." **Marianne**

"My life has changed so much. My boys come first. I don't have time to straighten my hair or do my make up most days. I make sure the boys are fine and ready before me. I don't care what I look like now. All my money goes on the boys and I hardly ever buy anything for me!" **Michelle**

"Being a mum puts everything into perspective - nothing else matters apart from protecting/caring/nurturing my children. I definitely love life more with children, coming from someone who always said "I didn't want any children." I can't imagine life without them now!" **Rachel**

"Motherhood has changed my priorities immeasurably and I'm a better person for it – I think?!" **Marika**

"I've changed a lot since having my baby; I'm one of the first of my friends. I miss going out. I miss the free time I had with my husband and my sense of working identity. On the positive side becoming a mother means I'm less worried about the small things - my focus is my daughter now. I can't believe I used to worry about half the things I did. I am in awe of all *mothers everywhere as it's such hard work. It has made me realise just what my mum did for me and my five (yes five!) siblings."* **Rebecca**

"In a lot of ways I don't think I have changed, I still feel like me but I have a completely different outlook on everything now. Some things just don't matter as much anymore. I find myself focusing on the bigger picture more not just the here and now. I am more inwardly confident in myself since having Grace - I'm not sure why really, maybe I'm still a bit proud of myself! My views have changed on a lot of things work being the biggest one, I always said I wouldn't stop work after my maternity leave but would like to go back part-time. When I got made redundant it changed everything as I quickly found out that I couldn't find another part-time job that paid enough so I had to get a full time job which I absolutely hated, I didn't think it would upset me quite so much from someone that used to really enjoy working. I now often feel resentful as it is taking my time away from being with Grace." **Samantha**

"My priorities have changed and I'm more grounded. I have a better sense of perspective. For example - I don't let work worry me anymore, or fret about seeing my friends as regularly as I used to... these things are important but they are not the priority. I say 'no' more these days whereas before I always said 'yes'! I'm a stronger and more determined person. I would never accept a situation that was unacceptable for my children in any area of my life. I am more aware of the world that we live in and the food we eat - I try to be a good role model and I want to protect them as much

as I can. All said though, I still have a strong sense of identity. I don't want to lose that. I don't ever want to feel as though I've totally lost 'me". **Liz**

"Although I am still career minded I love being with my children. I'd do anything for them. Anyone who worries about becoming a mother should try it. Don't let the thought of pain put you off - you forget about it soon after. It is hard work looking after children, but I don't know anyone that has every regretted it. I certainly don't." **Sandra**

Part Eight

Changes

And then there were three. How having a baby can alter a relationship...

As soon as you find out you're pregnant you change – and so does your partner. Suddenly he's not the most important thing in your life and some men struggle with this.

During your pregnancy you may feel very tired, not in the mood for sex or be struggling with sickness. In addition some women find their hormones are all over the place and they become tearful. The most important thing is to keep the lines of communication open and involve your partner as much as possible.

Also remember you are given a head-start in the bonding stakes because you're the one growing the baby – so you get a huge amount of time to get used to the idea. It's often harder for men. On that basis try to include your partner in the physical changes and what's happening at each stage to the baby. This will help him to feel involved and excited about what's happening.

Once the baby is born things change again. The sleepless nights, people coming round all the time and the general chaos of a newborn can be very disconcerting for many. Accept things will be different for a while but that you will soon find your own way and things will settle down. The early weeks are tough and can feel as though they'll go on forever but they won't. Before you know it you'll find your own rhythm and won't be able to imagine life without your little one.

During this time, take all the help that is offered to you and rest whenever you can. Try not to shut your partner out, include him where possible; tell him about your day and if you're struggling let him know.

Sometimes women moan when men won't offer help but then won't take help when it is being gifted. Also, let go of things being done perfectly – your partner will have his way of doing things, and that's okay. Try to relax, it really doesn't matter he's brought you a coffee using the best china or he didn't make the bed exactly the way you would - just go with it.

Because many men are by nature fixers he may also worry a lot more than your realise about the financial implications that the baby will have on you as a family. This is a real issue and something that needs to be discussed. If money is an issue let your partner know you're aware and that you're a team and will tighten your belts together.

An important thing to remember is that the baby is a by-product of your relationship and you and your partner are still entitled to have time together as a couple – even once the baby is born. If you're lucky enough to have parents who will have your baby/child/children overnight then let them go – time apart won't damage your child it will be good for you all – and think of the lie in!

It's well documented that a couple are most likely to separate when they have very young children – which is why it's important to keep the lines of communication open and to remind yourselves why you're together and chose to have a baby.

Try not to become one of those couples who only talk about their baby or child. Remember that one day your child will grow up and leave home and then you'll be left with your partner. Take time to nurture that relationship too – your child will thrive even more in a loving home, where people are kind to each other.

Remember that everything passes and this stage of your relationship won't last forever.

- Tips to nurture your relationship:
  - Talk, talk and talk some more
  - Make sure you involve your partner at every stage
  - If you're feeling unsupported – tell him. Men are not psychic
  - When you feel ready make sure you have some time as a couple
  - Try to think of things from your partner's perspective; if you're being snappy and short tempered imagine how that must be for him
  - Focus on the good things he does do – rather than constantly criticising him for the things he doesn't.

Relationship Changes by Psychotherapist, Eliott Green

"Being in relationship with another… whether as a wife, partner or friend involves an extension of the sense of self to encompass that of another. To not only acknowledge one's needs, but also to take another's into account. Additionally to take into account the relationship itself – the needs of the relationship i.e. 1 + 1 = 3 (self, other and relationship).

For example, I might want to go out and get stimulation. My partner might want a quiet night in. The relationship might be suffering from too much stimulation and not enough time to reflect and talk. It sounds as if a quiet night in might be in order.

Alternatively, we might have had a succession of quiet nights in and the relationship is suffering from boredom and apathy. It sounds as if doing something stimulating is called for.

On becoming a mother, the maths is once again called into question. From being in the one relationship, the next moment there are three relationships to consider. The original one you're in with your partner is added to by your new relationship with your child. Additionally there is also the relationship between your partner and their child to consider, the one which you are not directly a part of.

It is the sharing of these three relationships which most often poses challenges to the original relationship.

Some people only know how to put themselves first and find sharing almost intolerable. They often feel unloved and may end up looking for love outside of the relationship.

Others don't know how to put themselves first and find themselves torn by the conflicting needs of their partner and their baby. They often become overwhelmed and depressed.

Then there are the baby's needs to consider..."

© 2011 Eliott Green

It's a life changing event to have a baby – and the following women have shared some of the relationship highs and lows...

"It has quite a profound impact on your close relationships, not just with your partner but with friends and family members too. I remember my best friend at the time not taking to the news too well and suddenly I stopped getting invited to nights out. I wanted to scream 'I can still have a life!' People's perceptions of you change and they assume you don't have time for any social activity outside your new family bubble. The reality is you are quite often climbing the walls to escape for a bit of 'me' time!" **Jo**

"My husband and I are closer than ever. He was a great support and spoilt me in whatever way he could throughout my pregnancy (surprise bunches of flowers, meals out and attempted as best he could to be more help around the house)." **Emily**

"I didn't think having a baby would cause such a big change. I know I was naïve in the extreme! It does cause some marital strain I think; the wife feels like she has lost her independence and the man probably feels shut out - combine the two and you have a rather inflammatory cocktail of resentment, jealousy and total exhaustion." **Louise**

*"When I was pregnant with my daughter I had a very different idea of what having a baby would mean. I visualised lots of trips to the shops with my posh new pram looking at baby clothes, cooing over my little baby with my partner and keeping house. The reality was much harder. I had no idea how hard being a first

time mother was. My little girl had colic and literally slept or cried – and she didn't do a great deal of sleeping. I remember very clearly those early days and how it nearly drove my partner away. I was very realistic when I became pregnant for the second time. We both were - and I knew it would be hard but that the hard times end and you get a really great return at the end of all that effort." **Kelly**

"My husband was fantastic during my pregnancy. Sometimes, I would come home from work shattered and in pain from my hip. He would be my rock. Doing practical things like cooking dinner and going to the supermarket with me – pushing a trolley with SPD is not easy. He also was keen to be as involved as possible in the birth and preparing for it. He would do the maternity yoga with me at times, admittedly we would frequently end up in hysterics, but it meant that he knew what I was doing and what I would hopefully be doing during labour." **Caroline**

"Having a baby does change your relationship in many positive ways. Suddenly you are a family and there is a little person that every now and then you see a glimpse of one another in and it makes you smile. You are a team because everything you now do involves your new addition and you plan more together and worry more together about the right or wrong way to do things. As time goes by and you get used to your routines and it gets easier and you find a happy equilibrium. Making sure you spend time together alone is important too, having a 'date' night every now and then really takes the pressure off and lets you relax in each other's company again.

Inevitably you always talk about your baby but it's still nice to go out and not worry about the next feed or a dirty nappy." **Jo**

"My partner Roger has been a wonderful dad right from the beginning. During labour he was incredible – and I will never forget his face when the midwife handed him our first daughter Jessica – it's a picture that will stay in my mind always. Our girls are at school now but he's still just as hands on and gets as much out of them as I do. They're very lucky. Equally he supports me too – having the girls has bonded us as a family more than I dreamt it would." **Sandra**

"I will never forget finding out I was pregnant. My husband Nick and I had just got back from Sunday lunch at Café Rouge (I didn't realise at the time the glass of red wine with my lunch would be my last for a while!). I had bought a pregnancy test kit but was only a day or two late so hadn't taken a test yet, Nick was getting ready to go to golf and I decided to pop to the loo. When he came home later I was standing at the bottom of the stairs staring at the stick. When he asked if I was alright I gave him the stick, he looked at me and said 'Are you?' I said' Yes I think so,' I couldn't stop shaking. Nick was so happy, he couldn't stop grinning and hugging me. Nick was brilliant, and couldn't do enough for me. He was so excited to be a Daddy." **Samantha**

"My ex- husband Martin was very proud and enthusiastic throughout the whole experience. He was a massive support through the actual birth and helped me enormously by counting through the

contractions. He did fall asleep at one point but to be honest I did find that quite amusing. I think it's really tough on the partner. My memory of the first few hours after Billy's birth is not so positive though, as Martin left to go and ring people and sort out work issues. I was gutted by this, perhaps unreasonably so but I just didn't want to be alone and I wanted him there so much – but I don't think I actually told him that. Becoming a mum for the first time mum is hard and I would do many things differently. The over-riding thing is that I wish I had been stronger in communicating with my then-husband Martin. I wish I'd taken the time to share my thoughts, worries and frustrations. So many couples fall apart when the children come along and I'm sure people just don't realise what a strain having a child is on a relationship. People are very unprepared in this respect and it's a shame. I think the bottom line is lack of communication – I know that was certainly the case for us." **Liz**

"I can clearly remember and always will, sitting in the most beautiful square in a town in France, on what was meant to be a lovely last break for me and Ben before our son was due. I told Ben that I couldn't be with him anymore and that I didn't feel capable of being a mum and that maybe the baby would be better off if he was with his daddy and I had no involvement. An awful moment both in my life and pregnancy. I'm sure it was a complete moment of panic and realisation that my life was about to change forever. Ultimately, though Ben was the most amazing support I could have ever hoped for. He was supportive, loving, forgiving, thoughtful and cared so

much, even at the times when I was screaming, crying, feeling depressed, being hormonal and nasty to him. Despite his lack of household skills I couldn't wish for a better husband and having our children has made us so much stronger as a couple." **Tannita**

"The impact on your relationship is huge when you have a baby. I'm divorced from my first child's dad so when I was pregnant with my second child, it was my second husband's first child (keep up!). Because he's been in my life since Marley was young I think he thought he was prepared for having a baby. However, nothing prepares you for the tough first few months. No one copes well with little sleep but men are worse – even if they still get plenty. It's quite funny really as it becomes a competition as to who is most tired and who got more sleep. In the first three months I felt as though we were not in a relationship. We were existing. Every ounce of love and effort was going into our children, to the newborn and to her brother so he didn't feel rejected. It is amazing that you can do so much and put so much effort into your children all day every day. When they are both safely tucked up in bed you have nothing left to give each other. Finally, we have just started to spend a bit of quality time with each other and we talk more, mainly about how tired we are but still we talk!! You can't stop making an effort in your relationship especially after having children. The tough times do make your relationship stronger. Becoming parents is amazing and it is lovely to see how my partner is as a dad." **Amelia**

"I found I argued more with my partner at first about small things. Managing my time was suddenly a huge

priority. I kind of felt like I should be able to cope with all the housework, cooking, feeding the cat and looking after the baby as I was at home all day, but the reality is it is not always that easy. Things like my husband leaving the butter out the fridge would result in me freaking out and then crying that he didn't understand?! Dads are not going through the same crazy emotional changes that you and your body are. Sleep deprivation, hormones, juggling feeding, nappies, sleep times and making sure the dinner is on the table at the end of the day is pretty much an impossible feat... but we women do love a challenge and I learnt pretty quickly to give myself more of a break, nothing is really that important apart from you, your baby and your sanity. Leave the dusting to another day." **Joanne**

"Despite finding out my husband Dan was having an affair just a few weeks before I realised I was pregnant and us separating initially, having our second child Saskia has been the best thing that could have happened to our relationship. Dan had a lot of making up to do while I was pregnant but really came into his own and has been amazing ever since. We've made some changes as a family – I gave up a well paid job and am now working as a Teaching Assistant but I can honestly say we are a very happy family." **Tania**

"My wonderful husband was a massive support throughout my pregnancy and attended all the appointments. In labour he was there every step of the way and it's made me see him differently – even better." **Michelle**

Dr Pam Spurr Life Coach and relationship expert says you should expect the following 10 changes when a baby arrives

Sleepless Nights

Everyone warned how tired you'd be but you didn't expect full-on exhaustion. All the time.

Coping strategies:

- Always cat-nap when baby's napping
- Don't beat yourself up about not doing things such as ironing
- If breast-feeding, express milk so he can share night-feeds.

Lack of Time

Having a lie in and catching up with friends are distant memories. Your baby is a 24/7 way of life.

Coping strategies:

- Be queen of the quick catch-up – tell friends you are desperate to chat, but need to keep it brief
- Agree with your partner things you won't stress about for the first six months – like housework. Use that time for walks or watching DVDs – or get a cleaner if you can afford one.

Money Worries

They are only small but babies are money-munching machines.

Coping strategies:

- *Together make a list of outgoings and income. Get ruthless and look at anywhere you can save a few pounds*
- *Research online the best baby bargains*
- *Ask friends/family for hand-me-downs.*

Baby Talk

Conversations revolve completely around your baby. Of course the baby is mega-important but it's normal to long for some grown up chat.

Coping strategies:

- *It's vital you don't lose sight of focusing on each other*
- *Catch up on baby news from the day then ban further baby talk while catching up with each other*
- *Pull each other up if you slip back into baby stuff.*

Mood Swings

Fatigue and hormones mean that you're lovey dovey one moment, Cruella De Ville the next – tricky for your partner.

Coping strategies:

- *Try a daily meditation – take a few minutes to remind yourself you're doing your best*
- *Ask him for a massage – touch can be very soothing*
- *Avoid excess caffeine.*

Parenting Style

You love each other and had a baby together but that doesn't guarantee you'll agree on parenting techniques.

Coping strategies:

- *Find compromise between your points of view*
- *Alternate trying out each other's suggestions*
- *Don't turn differences into rows.*

In-Laws

These might already have been tricky but as grandparents they will stick their oar in and want to come over even more often.

Coping strategies:

- *Be fair in inviting grandparents over for equal time*
- *Agree to set boundaries on them interfering with baby techniques*
- *Show them your united front. They'll be less likely to butt in. Make them feel appreciated, asking for their advice when needed.*

Green-Eyed Monster

It's a shock when you realise he is jealous over the attention you give your child. But such complicated feelings are common.

Coping strategies:

- *If you suspect he feels this way, talk about it. Showing you recognise your attention is split in two will help*

- *Give him regular praise for the fantastic partner he is*
- *It only takes a moment to send him a quick text or email asking about him and his day.*

Baby Chores

Something as simple as nappy changing can cause big rows and divvying up chores can be challenging.

Coping strategies:

- *Make a list of baby chores. Split this logically. It might be easier for him to do the shopping and you do bath time*
- *Check often with each other if the chores-split is still working or if it needs adjustment.*

Sexy-time Sex – what's that?

You have distant memories of fancying each other but now there's barely a goodnight kiss.

Coping strategies:

- *Keep open about feelings towards restarting sex*
- *Depending on any pregnancy/birth complications ask your doctor's advice on restarting sex*
- *Rekindle romance first – be loving and affectionate*
- *Carve out 'couple time' the grandparents can babysit and swap babysitting with trusted friends.*

© 2011 Dr Pam Spurr

Part Nine

Getting me back

Because of the monumental, often shocking changes that a woman goes through after having a baby it's only natural that you can't wait to get 'me' back. That's totally normal and it doesn't mean that you're not a good mum because you'd quite like to be able to have a wee or a drink in peace.

As soon as possible, I'd suggest taking some time out for yourself – even if it is just for ten minutes every day. See if you can pencil in a daily time-slot where your partner can take over - and then leave them to it. Don't hover in the background – go and enjoy your precious 'me time'.

Thing to try:

- Run a bath, light a candle and immerse yourself in a little slice of heaven
- Read a magazine, the trashier the better
- Speak to a friend/family member – someone who will listen and understand the good and bad days ideally
- Write in your journal. Sometimes expressing how you feel makes you feel so much better – it's the act of releasing that is very cleansing and if you've had a great day it's nice to keep a record for the future
- Go for a walk and savour the fact that for the duration you have your hands to yourself
- Do some yoga or Pilates. Stretching for just ten minutes a day will help you enormously and it will release some feel good chemicals to boot.

Exercise

Most women are eager to get back into shape once their baby is born – one thing I always say to the postnatal mums I teach is to remember that it took nine months to grow the baby and for your body to change – so give yourself time to get back to your best.

Yes some women are lucky and leave their hospital in their pre-pregnancy skinny jeans but most don't – especially if like me you put on a lot of weight while you were expecting.

It's important not to over-do exercise or to go on a crazy crash diet – you'll only end up bingeing in secret and feeling guilty, or getting poorly. Just begin by making small lifestyle changes and gradually you will lose excess weight.

Once Zak was born and I was able to I couldn't wait to start exercising again. I've always been so active and I found the limitations during pregnancy difficult. I put on a lot of weight when I was expecting, and although I lost an awful lot after he was born (a lot of it was water) I needed to tone up.

I'd qualified to teach yoga so I began doing that every day and I also joined a Buggyfit group and for me that was great. Walking is probably one of the best things you can do with your little one – not only are you both getting lots of fresh air but it's the perfect time to chatter away to your baby or sing songs. You may look a bit crazy, but that's okay. If you can get out for 20 minutes every day you'll feel so much better and your little one will thrive with all the fresh air.

As and when you want to do more take it easy and listen to your body at every stage. If something doesn't feel right – it's probably because it isn't.

The ACOG (American Congress of Obstetricians and Gynaecologists, 1994) recommend that women should avoid all physical stress for two weeks – this means you're not to carry anything heavier than the baby. Full daily activities shouldn't be resumed until six weeks and if you've delivered by caesarean section a woman shouldn't exercise for 12 weeks after delivery to allow proper healing time. It is important, after giving birth to be cleared by your doctor before you start any new regime and remember to be realistic. If you've spent nine months sitting around eating cream cakes you're going to find any exercise difficult at first, but stick with it and it will get easier week-by-week.

The benefits of postnatal exercise include:

- Improved posture
- Increased muscle strength and tone
- Increased stamina and energy
- Increased weight loss and improved body imaged
- Increased self-confidence
- Reduced anxiety.

It may take six weeks for muscles to fully recover or even longer if they were weak before pregnancy. Gentle abdominal exercises in the early postnatal period will help enormously. To strengthen your tummy muscles begin with your pelvic floor exercises and additionally tighten your tummy at the same time. These can be commenced immediately after birth. I always suggest to the postnatal women I teach to try and find a slot in the day when you can do your pelvic floor exercises in peace. Feeding your little one is the ideal time.

First six weeks

Walking is the best exercise you can do, and it doesn't cost a penny. Hopefully taking your baby out for a stroll is a big motivator for you. If you try to do a combination of walking every day as well as doing your pelvic floor exercises that will be enough.

After your six week check

Once you've been signed off by the doctor and as long as you're feeling strong enough try to increase your exercise regime – but still be sensible. I wouldn't advise a hard core body attack, spinning or step class for a while. If you do any classes, whether at a gym, local hall or community centre you must tell the instructor you've recently had a baby so they can make any relevant adaptations.

Try the following:

Walking – increase your distance and pace now. If you want to do some more buy some ankle or wrist weights that will add a bit of resistance training to your walk. There are lots of buggy based exercise groups out there where you go for a walk with other women and do some specific exercises on the way, such as lunges, squats and tricep dips. It's a great way to meet new mums as well as toning up your body.

Yoga – try a postnatal class initially and then a 'normal' class but be aware you may not be as strong as you were so take it easy. Be conscious of not over-stretching in class or competing with other students.

Pilates – is great for re-gaining your core strength and also brilliant for strengthening your back which is often weakened after birth.

Swimming – being in the water is lovely – as long as you feel confident in your swimming costume. Try to swim for a minimum of 20 minutes each time. Swimming is great for your tummy and also one of the best exercises you can do for your back.

Aqua natal – if you enjoy swimming try an aqua natal class or if they don't do one in your area a normal aqua aerobics class will be fine after your six week check.

As you get stronger you can increase your exercise – but do be aware that if you over-do it in the early days there's a risk of hurting yourself and then not being able to do anything.

Food

Remember if you're breast-feeding you will need an extra 500 calories each day. If possible try to get these extra calories out of healthy food rather than a Mars bar.

If you want to lose some weight rather than cutting out whole food groups your best bet is to eat three well-balanced meals a day, drink lots of water and limit your in-take of too much sugar or fat.

Making the most of your looks

Okay, so you may be a few pounds heavier, with dark shadows under your eyes but you can still make the most of yourself. If you wash your hair every day and apply even a bit of make-up you'll feel much better for it. There's nothing like a bit of bronzer to lift your spirits!

Personally it's important for me that I've showered and done my hair every day and put on some foundation. I just feel like me when my hair and make-up is done and I don't scare myself when I catch sight of myself in the mirror. When Zak was tiny I'd put him in his cot for a while and let him play for a few minutes while I had a much deserved shower. On the occasional bad day if I thought he wouldn't settle he came into the bathroom with me in his baby seat and watched me washing. Where there's a will there's a way!

Many women really come into themselves as they get older and having a baby gives many a sense of confidence they've never had before which shows in their faces. If however, you're not happy with the face that greets you when you look in the mirror there are things you can do;

Beauty Editor Lauren Naylor gives her top-tips for new mums

Eyes

They say the eyes are the window to the soul, therefore your lashes are the window pane and in charge of 'opening them up'. The first tell-tale sign you are absolutely shattered, is through your eyes.

Even if you don't have time for anything else, wear mascara or even get your eyelashes tinted at your local salon to save precious minutes each morning.

For fresh and awake eyes, use white eyeliner along your waterline (inside the rim). The white instantly gives a clearer iris and can help conceal tell-tale redness, making eyes look visibly fresher and younger.

Glow givers

If you're very dehydrated and tired wrinkles will be more visible, so ensure your skin is always hydrated from the inside out by drinking eight glasses of water per day and moisturising your face thoroughly every morning and evening.

If your skin is in need of a pick-me-up try facial oil at night and allow it to work its magic while you (hopefully) sleep! Facial oil isn't just for dry skin, it's actually good for oily too, as it works to regulate sebum production.

Baby borrower

Yes! Your baby's products can double up for you. While you are rubbing moisturiser into your baby's skin or massaging them borrow some of their bottom butter for your face or hands.

Waitrose's Baby Bottom Butter which is under £3 made the headlines when it sold a 14-year supply in just 12 months. The fabulous cream works as a facial moisturiser, hand cream and will sort out any dry spots like elbows and knees.

If you haven't had time to wash your hair - shake some baby talc into the roots to soak up grease – it will cut through oily roots and turn your lank locks into lustrous ones - perfect if mum-in-law pays a surprise visit.

Vaseline is also an amazing multi-tasking product slicking eyebrows into place, or even in replacement of mascara. Ease it from root to tip of your eyelash to give them a glossy - no-make up finish. You can also slick Vaseline onto your cheekbones to give you a dewy-look, or even use it as an eye make-up remover - it works fabulously!

And of course don't forget your Johnson's heroes such as baby lotion and baby shampoo. They are all mum-friendly too - who doesn't love the saccharine sweet scent of baby products?

Clothes

Erica Davies is Executive Fashion Editor at the Sun and has her own style blog, modernmummusthave.com, a Fashion Editor's guide to life, style and kids.

She is also a mum, with a two-year old toddler and a month old baby. Here, Erica shares her top style secrets

No one can deny that having a baby is one of the most exciting things that can happen to you.

But while you are coming to terms with this little gurgling bundle of joy, you also have to deal with the after-math of pregnancy and childbirth.

Oh and did we mention the sleep deprivation?

Needless to say, unless you are a total anomaly and did not put on an inch during your pregnancy, your body will have changed. Massively.

Whether you have gone up one size or three, are dealing with new body issues and sore boobs, post-childbirth dressing can be just as challenging as looking after your baby.

In between feeds and nappy changes, you want to feel good about yourself. It isn't easy, but a few clever tips will see you ditch the oversized pyjama bottoms before you know it.

And it really won't take long until you are back in the style saddle – honestly.

Don't be too fast to ditch your maternity wear

You won't need them forever, but don't be too quick to dump your pregnancy gear in the charity shop.

The stretch skinny jeans, maternity leggings and button-up tops and tunics you wore during your pregnancy will all be life savers in the first few weeks, when you really won't know what has hit you and you definitely don't want to be worrying about outfits.

Plus, when your body feels as though it belongs to someone else, you will feel comfortable in them at least.

Get properly measured for bras

It is so important to get properly measured for bras after your milk has come in. Whether you will be breast feeding or not, your boobs will take on a life of their own for a few weeks.

Being comfortable in practical, well-fitting nursing bras really will make a huge difference.

Try not to be put off by some of the prices, which can be expensive. Two bras that fit properly and support your new-size boobs are all you need - and they really are an investment.

Think about night time comfort too. Sleep bras are a must as you will probably be leaking and need to wear breast pads for a few months. These too will offer your boobs the support they need.

And take a tip from the celebrities – try wearing control pants to pull you in and start toning up you tum again. Gwyneth Paltrow admitted to wearing two pairs post-birth at all times.

Think capsule

Don't pick up where you left off. Your life- and style - has totally changed.

Take a good look at your figure. Unless you are one of the very lucky ones, you have probably gone up a size or two during your pregnancy and are now a bit softer around the middle.

Be honest with yourself. There is no shame in buying a pair of size 16 jeans if they are the most flattering and comfortable.

Realise that you won't be this size forever and that you just want to have a few decent wardrobe options while you adjust to motherhood and your new body.

Making it easy should be your buzz words, so a capsule wardrobe in a few colours will mean your clothes will work hard mixing and matching.

Choose layers, so think about a vest top underneath a tunic or blouse and a scarf for your top half.

If you are breastfeeding, easy access is required and you do not want to feel too restricted in jumpers or high-necks. A scarf also doubles up as a discreet feeding shield if you are out and about.

Sludgy shades of inky blue, grey and khaki green always look chic and timeless and mix well together. A brightly patterned scarf will pull the look together perfectly.

Returning to me

Little by little you will become your old self again – a slightly altered, battle weary version perhaps but you nonetheless. As your baby grows older your child-free days will seem like a distant, hazy memory – something you look back on occasionally with a mixture of longing and shock. Longing that you used to be able to lie in bed regularly until 10.00am and shock that you were so selfish, opinionated –and well different.

Enjoy your journey into motherhood and the changes along the way – acknowledge them and accept that you are now a mother – before all else.

There will be times when you yearn for your old life and if things do feel too much then take a break if you can. You are still entitled to some free time without a little one attached to you and sometimes a break away from your child when you get the chance to miss them is a really good thing as when you return to each other you'll both be fresh and eager to be together again.

You don't have to be with your child 24/7 to be a good mum – but equally if you make the choice never to be parted from your little one that is up to you.

Before too long you'll get your body and yourself back. Remember the woman you were before and allow her to put in an appearance even if it's only sometimes, so you don't feel as though you've been lost along the way.

Acknowledge the things that make you feel good, whether it's reading a book, or sharing a bottle of red with a girlfriend and try to do them as often as you can. Just because you're a mum it doesn't mean you have to sacrifice yourself entirely. In my experience the women that are happiest are not those with all the money and resources, but who make a little time for themselves. It's about managing your time effectively and accepting help as and when it's offered. Don't make the mistake of always being at the bottom of the list and simmering inside with resentment. It won't do you or your baby any good in the long run.

What you do to feel good

> *"I make sure I go to the gym at least twice a week, whether it's for a run or to a class. That time away from home is really important and I feel better for it."* **Liz**
>
> *"I have monthly reflexology sessions at home. The way I look at it I don't drink or smoke and it's my treat and keeps me sane."* **Felicity**
>
> *"I meet up with friends regularly and share a bottle (or two) of wine. It's important to have time away from the children, no matter how much I love them."* **Ava**
>
> *"I've joined a book club and it's been a revelation. Not only have I started reading again which I had neglected since having children – but I really look forward to our meetings where we talk about something totally different from the children."* **Louise**

Women are often guilty of trying to do it all and here, best-selling author Giselle Green and mum of six boys shares her top ten tips on finding me-time

1. Delegate

Kids love coming home from school and jumping straight on the computer, games console or TV. If it drives you round the bend that they aren't helping out round the house, get them into the habit of seeing 'computer time' or 'TV time' as a reward (for helping you).

Start by only letting them on the computer after helping you with a chore. They'll soon be queuing up to clear those dishes.

2. Make it fun

Whatever you need doing, get the whole family interested and involved by having fun. Even things like redecorating needn't be a chore - kids love pulling down wallpaper. When their bedrooms look like a pigsty, hold a competition to see who can fill a bin-bag or the laundry basket first.

If you're trying to get them to tidy their rooms promise them a game of twister or a board game in their bedroom - but only once the floor of their bedroom is completely toy-free!

3. Teach them as they help

Even little ones can be encouraged into things like sock pairing - this involves colour and size-sorting and it's educational too. The same goes for putting groceries away after a shopping trip. One child can put away the frozen food, or tins and packets in cupboards. This is not only great for saving you time, but it shows that what they eat doesn't get conjured up out of 'nowhere', so it teaches them appreciation too.

4. Get your man on-board

Arguments and discussions about the right way to do things waste valuable energy and time. It's no good you laying down rules that the other one doesn't stick to. This will only cause problems like, 'Daddy always lets me sit in the front of the car and you won't', or 'Mum always lets me have biscuits before bedtime'.

Agree on boundaries with your partner and stick to them - the time saved by having to talk about it afterwards can be used for a little me-time.

5. Agree a deal

Why not trade a weekend away on your own or with your girlfriends in exchange for your partner doing the same? You'll come back refreshed and revitalised and when it's your other-half's turn - so will they! If you don't have a partner to share the children with, try kid-swapping weekends with friends. But however you do it, get that time away.

Just make sure you're happy with who you leave them with, as you don't want to spend your time away from them worrying!

6. Know what you want

Make a list of 'time-treats' - little things that you know you'd love to do for yourself if only the day were long enough. A 10-minute time-treat might be sitting down and reading a magazine or a couple of chapters in a book, a 30-minute time-treat might see you catching up on your favourite soap (if you've got two week's worth recorded you're never going to catch up otherwise!). This way when free time does crop up, you'll know exactly what you want to do and won't waste it.

7. Ask for 'me-time' as a present

If you've got a birthday round the corner and people ask what you'd like, don't be afraid to suggest something that little bit different. Maybe you've always fancied going to London to have a treatment at a well-known hairstylist? Or you want to go out for a meal with friends instead of doing the cooking. It's important to try and carve out that little space in the day that's especially for you.

8. Beware the time thieves

We all love chatting with friends, but there are always people who keep you talking that little bit longer than they should do, certain parents outside the school gates, people in shopping queues or colleagues at work who eat into your time when you don't really mean them too.

Imagine you're on a 'time-wasting diet' where hanging about for too long listening to other people's moans is the same as a calorie-packed doughnut!

9. Don't do what you don't really have to do

Have you found yourself ironing shirts that were only going to be worn under jumpers, or sweeping leaves that were only going to pile up again? Well don't. Some women find it impossible to stop and the minute a chance comes to relax they ignore it and look for the next task.

If this sounds like you, then slow down. Look for the gaps and spaces where you can get away without being so busy and use some of that for a bit of me-time.

10. Make it count

We all know kids are exhausting but they grow up unbelievably quickly, meaning that your chances to build special memories together don't last all that long. The key is to find something that counts as quality time for both parent and child. Something as simple as a bike ride in the country can suffice. Just make sure you're fitting in quality time for everyone.

© 2010 **Giselle Green**

Part Ten

Perfect Mums

In recent years the pressure on women and mothers in particular has undoubtedly increased. Everything from your weight, clothes and the pram you push is scrutinised – there is pressure, pressure and yet more pressure on us all.

I can never, ever remember my own mum lambasting herself over the decisions she made about her parenting style and I know when I speak to other friends their parents didn't either.

Now, we're constantly bombarded with this report that report and every other report about the right way to do it but the thing is nobody seems to agree on what that right way is.

The end result is many women feel inadequate and as though they're the only ones not blending organic carrots and doing five stimulating baby groups a day and then when they're older doing advanced French at the age of five and Mandarin at 15. It's all too much.

If only women and mothers could be more honest and admit they too have hard days and make mistakes instead of putting on a front that everything in their world is perfect.

The constant images of celebrities looking effortlessly groomed and slender within days of having a baby is enough to make you want to leap back into bed and stay there forever.

Just remember these women have huge amounts of money, status, staff – and they're paid to look like that (even if it's inadvertently). So embrace CBeebies and the odd jar of baby food. Here's to a new breed of more relaxed, contented mums which surely leads to more relaxed, contented babies.

It's funny the things that stick in your mind when you're expecting and I think that we need to remember that pregnant women, especially when they're expecting their first child are pretty vulnerable.

There are so many books and authority figures saying this is right and that is right that it's very difficult to know what to do - is it wrong to let my baby cry? Will I cause my child problems forever if he does/doesn't have a dummy? It's so confusing.

I read a well-known baby book when I was 16 weeks pregnant. A friend bought it for me when I told her my baby news. I eagerly went to bed that night with my new book and just cried. It was so regimented that I knew it wouldn't ever work for me and I actually thought that was what I had to do if I wanted my baby to thrive. The author was so insistent in her words that I felt that if I didn't do it that way I would fail in my role as a mother from day one.

Luckily I have since learnt that it's okay to trust your instincts and I didn't need such a rigid routine with my baby anyway.

However, I did do strange things looking back. When Zak was first born I had read somewhere it was best for a baby to be fed in the same place at every feed. So for the first few weeks of his life I sat on a wooden chair up in his nursery for hours at a time while nursing him. Then one day it dawned on me that I didn't have to do that and in fact it would probably be better for him to see some different furnishings.

I've spoken to some mums who have confided there were certain beliefs they had before they became a mum that didn't last long once they realised in the grand scheme of things some of their rigid beliefs really didn't matter.

Here, some mums share how they altered their expectations once their baby was born…

"I put so much pressure on myself to breastfeed and really struggled with it at first which made the situation even worse. As soon as I relaxed and just accepted it might not be right for my baby I had success and I was able to breastfeed my baby until she was six months." **Ava**

"I wanted everything to be just so and didn't factor in that being a mum at home with your new baby is tough – without the added pressure of having a perfect house and a fresh home-cooked meal on the table every evening. Our house turned into a pressure pot waiting to explode until I took a step back and cut myself some slack." **Jo**

"I'd made a pact with myself that I wouldn't ever give my baby a jar or packet food. I had it in my mind that people who used convenience foods with their babies were just lazy. Well that lasted for about two weeks. Every time I went anywhere I had countless Tupperware pots of food with me before it dawned on me that it didn't matter if my child had the odd jar – the annoying thing was that he preferred the ready-made stuff too!" **Clare**

"TV! I thought we'd have none, but I have since decided that an hour or two a day is not the end of the world, especially when we have 'earned' it by taking the dog out or something." **Amber**

"I swore I'd never give my kids sweets but as they got older I just realised it wasn't realistic as sweets are all around them and I didn't want them to be different to other children or become secret binge-eaters! I also hated guns and was adamant my children would never have toy guns, until I found them sitting eating their lunch aged two and four, shaping their sandwiches into guns and shooting each other!" **Shelley**

"I've always hated dummies and promised myself my children wouldn't ever have them until I'd had a few sleepless nights and would have given them anything to help them sleep! Enter the dummy. I was strict with it and only used them for naps and they both gave them up by the time they were two – I really don't know what I was worried about." **Marika**

"Biscuits. I remember getting totally furious when despite asking her not to, my mother-in-law gave my daughter a biscuit! I stewed on it for weeks. Five years on I totally accept – and love that Nanny has a special biscuit box for the kids when they visit here. Everyone is happy and really... a couple of biscuits isn't the end of the world!" **Tamandra**

Something I've learnt along the way is not to judge other mums for the way they're bringing up their children. I'm a bit of a believer in, 'There but for the grace of God...' None of us are perfect and there's no such thing as a perfect child. It could just as easily be you dealing with a screaming toddler in the supermarket as some other poor woman. It doesn't mean she's a bad mother or has a particularly horrible or naughty child – it's just a bad moment, and we all have them.

We all have our issues with our children and just because you have a child who sleeps through the night it doesn't mean there's not another area that you don't struggle with.

There have been moments when I have been mortified by Zak's behaviour and felt so embarrassed that he's reduced me to tears. I know when I've spoken to other mums they've had their moments too and knowing that is a massive relief.

Here, some other mums share their thoughts on perfection and what it means to them

"I used to strive to be the perfect mum, perfect wife and perfect employee. As I've got older I've realised doing your best under the circumstances, whatever they may be at any given time is enough. And I'm not sure perfection exists. One person's idea of a perfect mum may be quite different to another's. The pressure comes from society which judges everyone. It comes from peers, health visitors, from family, schools and the government – and I think as children grow older, from the children themselves, "so- and-so's mum does this, buys that, gives lifts..." No wonder we're all exhausted. **Shelley**

"I used to worry about what everyone thought of how I parented my girls. Was it right? Was it wrong? Was my child's behaviour a result of good or bad parenting? Now... I don't give a damn what other people think. I do my very best, I think what I do is right at that moment in time. People that have children that are 'so well behaved' and look down on others having difficulties watch out. It hits us all at some point. I have children, aged, 13, 11, seven and four. One constantly gives me grief and one never

does – but I remain open minded and wait for the day she does! Each child brings their own challenges for me to overcome! As a parent you never stop being challenged with a new problem or situation. We are all constantly learning." **Abi**

"I think we feel we should be a perfect parent because we want a perfect child. But they don't read the perfect child manual before they are born! I think we need to throw the books and ideals away and bring them up how our instinct tells us, after all we are all individuals and we know instinctively what is right for OUR child – but it isn't necessarily right for other people's children." **Fraz**

"It's very tough being a new mum. I struggled to get a shower some days – let alone getting the house tidy and the washing done. I think we pile pressure on ourselves because people always want to visit and we feel we should have the house spic and span and look polished, even though it really doesn't matter. I've learnt to be a lot more chilled since having my little girl but still feel I'd like to do more, just for me though, not anyone else!" **Gemma**

"I do feel pressure, but more from myself than anyone else. I want to be the best mum I can to my children. I increasingly worry less what other people think of my parenting skills and think more about how happy my children are. I now feel very comfortable in my parenting. I think I'm a pretty good mum – but certainly not perfect. Who wants perfection anyway? It's boring." **Marika**

"Pressure comes from not only media but also family who have strong views on how children should behave and the like. I think that pressure can also come from not wanting to repeat perceived negative parts of your own childhood (futile effort!)." **Tamandra**

"If we were perfect there would be nothing left to learn, nothing to strive for and no sense of achievement or fulfilment. By openly accepting our flaws and working to improve and grow, we teach our kids a valuable lesson. (Note to self... repeat several times a day until it sinks in!)." **Paula**

One More Step Along the World I Go...

Enjoy the journey as you grow from a woman into a mother. Revel in the good days, learn from the bad ones and above all don't put too much pressure on yourself. Just be as good as you can at any given time.

There will be times when you feel as though you're being pushed to the end of your limits and in these moments you are allowed to go into a room by yourself and scream and shout as much as you need to.

Accept the mistakes you make along the way and trust you learn far more from your errors. Nobody gets it right all the time and it's pointless trying to. You're just setting yourself up to fail if perfection is your goal. Don't beat yourself up about the choices you make – guilt has to be the most worthless emotion there is. If you're not happy with something do what you can to change it rather than spending time wallowing.

Show your child you love them with all your heart and remember to show love to yourself too.

Ultimately love is the only thing that matters and if you tell your child every day you love them and show it too they'll forgive you when you mess up just as we forgive our children their misdemeanours.

Enjoy your baby as the days pass in a flash and before you know it you won't be the person they'll turn to when they fall but then you'll know you've done your job well as they go on with their lives as an independent person knowing in their hearts they had a mum who did her best, from the moment of birth and beyond.

Thank you and all the best to you and your family.

If you've got a birth story to share please contact me at
www.frombumptobabybook.co.uk

GLOSSARY

ACUPUNCTURE

www.acupuncture.org.uk

www.emmacannon.co.uk

AROMATHERAPY

www.aromatherapycouncil.org

BABY MASSAGE

www.iaim.org.uk The IAIM is a non-profit organisation founded in 1986. The IAIM mission statement is 'to promote nurturing touch and communication through training, education and research so that parents, caregivers and children are loved, valued and respected throughout the world community.'

BABYCENTRE

www.babycentre.co.uk the UK's number own pregnancy and parenting website full of tips and information for mums-to-be and families.

BIRTHLIGHT

www.birthlight.com Focuses on a holistic approach to pregnancy, birth and babyhood using yoga and breathing methods.

BREASTFEEDING

www.abm.me.org Association of Breastfeeding Mothers

BUGGY WORKOUTS

Working out with your baby in its buggy is genius. There are several companies around the country;

www.buggyfit.co.uk

www.buggypower.co.uk

CRYING BABIES

www.cry-sis.org.uk Cry-Sis support site for those with crying, sleepless and demanding babies and children.

DOULA

www.doula.org.uk

HOMEBIRTHS

www.homebirth.org.uk

www.birthchoiceuk.com

INDEPENDENT MIDWIFE

www.independentmidwives.org.uk

MASSAGE

www.gcmt.org.uk The GCMT is the governing body for massage therapies and bodyworks and soft tissue techniques in the UK.

NATIONAL INSTITUTE FOR HEALTH & CLINICAL EXCELLENCE

www.nice.org.uk National Institute for Health & Clinical Excellence

NATIONAL CHILDBIRTH TRUST

www.nctpregnancyandbabycare.com

NETMUMS

www.netmums.com covers everything you could ever need as a pregnant woman or as a mum. There is information on groups, campaigns and opinions galore.

NURSERY EQUIPMENT

www.babychild.org.uk nursery furniture, maternity wear, baby, toddler and children's lifestyle and health products.

OSTEOPATHY

www.osteopathy.org.uk

PREPMYBABY

www.prepmybaby.co.uk an online store which aims to provide mums with the most stylish, functional and value for money, mum and baby products.

REFLEXOLOGY

www.aor.org.uk

RELATIONSHIP HELP AND ADVICE

www.drpam.co.uk

ROYAL COLLEGE OF OBSTETRICIANS AND GYNAECOLOGISTS

www.rcog.org.uk

SPINNING BABIES

www.spinningbabies.com lots of information about positioning for the baby and poses to try to get baby into the best birth post possible

STYLE

www.modernmummusthave.com Fashion Editor Erica Davies shares her fashion and style tips

SURE START

www.direct.gov.uk/surestart UK Government initiative with the aim of giving children the best possible start if life through improvement of childcare, early education, health and family support. There are groups all over the country.

YOGA

www.yogaalliance.co.uk

www.bwy.org.uk

www.birthlight.co.uk